"A SHOT IN THE ARM"

by

Malcolm C. McDonald, OAM.

This treatise tells of the history of the first 100 Years of the QATB with anecdotes of the life of an Ambulance Officer and the introduction of intravenous cannulation.

It covers the establishment of the (QAS), Queensland Ambulance Service in 1991 and a brief on the next 25 years to 2016.

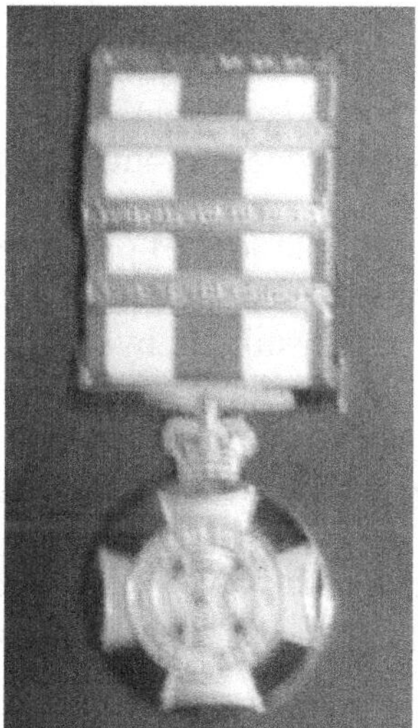

"A SHOT IN THE ARM"

COVER PIECE: 1991 Multi vehicle accident within the Ipswich District.

The Emergency Team of Police, Fire Brigade and QATB Ipswich Ambulance in attendance.
Superintendent McDonald attended as Site Commander with Medical Officer from IGH – the red helmets denote their position.

Patients required Pre-hospital Emergency Care for multiple trauma, monitoring for cardiac abnormalities and intravenous cannulation for fluid replacement.

ISBN: 978-0-9751966-4-9 First Edition 2016
Published by McDonald Books
121 / 8 George Street, Caboolture, Q. 4510.
Email: malmcdon@westnet.com.au

Respect is extended to persons involved as recorded in press, agreed training exercises, official or diary reports – E&OE.

"A SHOT IN THE ARM" is the euphemism to recognise the sensibilities of certain groups of the 21st century, rather than: "The invasive technique of inserting a large bore Needle into a Vein in the Arm"

This treatise tells of the history of the first 100 Years of the QATB with anecdotes of the life of an Ambulance Officer and the changing role over the decades to the introduction of intravenous cannulation.

It shares insights into the first days of the (QAS), Queensland Ambulance Service in 1991 with a brief on Executives and on qualifications and medical techniques over the next 25 years to 2016 and involves members of three generations who served.

It is the 2016 sequel to *the1993 "TRUST ME – I'M AN AMBULANCE OFFICER" which has been reviewed and updated due to numerous requests.*

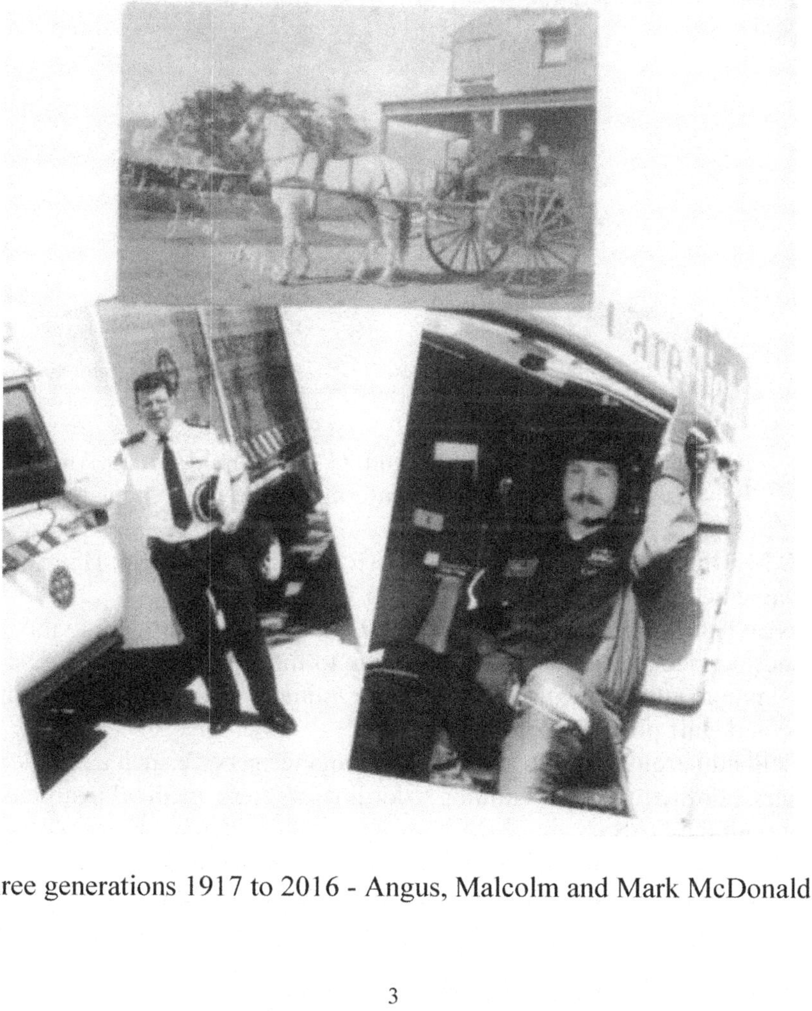

Three generations 1917 to 2016 - Angus, Malcolm and Mark McDonald.

The three generations:
Angus McDonald the father of the author was a Bearer at Rockhampton Centre and transferred from there to the QATB Cairns in 1917.
In 1918 the Cairns Brigade purchased a 1918 Hupmobile and Angus McDonald "being a competent Motor Driver was placed in charge of the new vehicle."

Malcolm C. McDonald, OAM, FPA., joined the Queensland Ambulance Service in 1959 as an Honorary Officer at QATB Cairns, then as a permanent Officer at Julia Creek in 1962 and to Rockhampton Centre in 1964 where he also served as an Aerial Ambulance Attendant in the Central Qld. Aerial Ambulance.
Appointed Supt. of Wowan Centre in 1969 then Maleny Centre and to Gatton Centre in 1973, Ipswich 1979. Assistant Commissioner Region 5, Brisbane 1991.

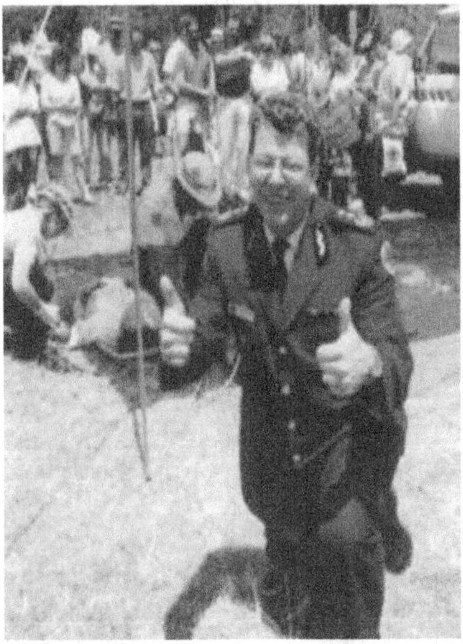

Assistant Commissioner Malcolm C. McDonald, FIAO(Aust).
Pre-hospital Emergency Care International Conference -1992.

Mark C. McDonald, ASM. Dip. Mgt; BN(RN); BHS; Adv. Dip. HSc (Intensive Care Paramedic) ; Ass. Dip. App. Sc. (Amb.).
Joined as an Honorary Ambulance officer 1975 before appointment to the Ambulance service as a Paramedic, advancing to Intensive Care Paramedic and later progressing into staff education as the Senior Clinical Educator (Post Graduate program) and staff professional development.
He has held numerous positions with the Ambulance service such as Regional Education Coordinator, State Training Coordinator, Aero-medical instructor and Assessor with the QAS.
Mark was awarded the Ambulance Service Medal, ASM, in 2015 and currently holds the position of Assistant Superintendent, Manager Clinical Education, Metro South LASN, Queensland Ambulance Service, Spring Hill. Qld. 2016.

PROLOGUE:

In the transient electronic world of today is there time for contemplation!

Might a Paramedic in the frenzied time slot of today wonder as to how their counterpart operated 120 years ago when a sweaty horse had to be rubbed down after a case before handwriting all details for records.

- Did the advances of 'today' just 'happen' over one long week-end?
- Is there anything of value to be learned or anything treacherous to avert?
- Or is it just "it's cool man, let's move on."

We touch on past practice to appreciate the escalation of progress in the cultural, educational and industrial systems from the 1890s to the 1990s -
Ice chests to computer controlled refrigerators – wood stoves to microwave ovens – helium passenger balloons to jet powered Airbus and Spacecraft to Mars – crystal sets to satellite communication – a wooden peg leg to SS prosthesis with articulated joint and assisted function – deafness to bionic hearing – sketch maps to satellite navigation systems – hand written notes to instant computer data and reporting.

The list is endless. These were all discovered/ invented/ manufactured by people of the twentieth century.

In this treatise we address the influence of such systems through the lives of Ambulance officers in the environment of the 20th and 21st century.

The history of the 100 years of the QATB and a brief on the 25 years of the QAS to July 2016.

DEDICATION:

To my family, my wife Val and Mark, David and Annette, who are every part of my life and shared my career.

ACKNOWLEDGMENTS :

Success in any major endeavour requires commitment which demands sacrifice of personal interests and time but there must be a balance between professional demand and family responsibility.

Fortunately as the Superintendent my residence was within the Centre complex which provided family stability but automatically included the family within the Ambulance fraternity.

The support by my wife and family provided a solid base for my career.

Dr. Wilson – a dedicated local Doctor who recognised sincere interest and endeavour and supported this by encouraging further study.

Medical Profession – most members of the Medical profession were generous with their advice and instruction, ever willing to assist and give of their time.

Position - I was alone but not lonely– I enjoyed the confidential, at times intricate planning required to foil retractors when initiating a controversial and innovative program and to work within the system to maintain the integrity of assessment and certification.

The Ambulance fraternity – to be part of a profession which attracts people of like commitment to 'do that bit more' and who have a connection to the sensitivity of all people, and with that touch of courage and drama which describes 'the Ambulance Officer,' is an honour.

INTRODUCTION.

Ambulance Paramedics and officers of the 21st century who were born about 1970 would have little idea of the everyday life of the populace and the structure of the Queensland Ambulance Transport Brigade in the early years so will have little conception of the standard of Medical provision of those times nor of the accepted and respected administration of Ambulance services by the Q.A.T.B.

We will relate the circumstance of that period as a point of appreciation and understanding of the evolution of our service.

This treatise provides a brief preliminary overview of the early years from 1892 of the QATB and sets the period comparisons of the progression in Pre-hospital Patient Care to WWI, to post WWII, in PART ONE.

We provide anecdotes in the daily experiences of the Ambulance officer in an easy manner for general understanding with some traditional advice from experience.

PART TWO addresses the vision and commitment in the late 20th century to have Health authorities recognise and introduce life saving procedures for fluid replacement from the onset at scene by certified Ambulance Officers.

This records the evolution of training to1982 when Ipswich Ambulance initiated the pass/fail criteria of knowledge and skills for the appointment of certified Senior Officers by 1983.

It provides the history of, and lists the development of certified procedures for Ambulance Officers to administer intravenous cannulation and infusion at scene by 1985, and the establishment of the pathway for this to be accepted by the QATB and later by the QAS in 1991.

Part Two: *this narration is in a chronological context.*
The establishment of the state Queensland Ambulance Service, (QAS), in 1991 and a brief on the escalation of academic qualifications from Associate Diploma, to Diploma and then to Degree with relevant case histories of 1989 and in 2013.

There is an enlightening article on the first days of the QAS from 1st July 1991 followed by profiles of the QAS management.

The Appendix outlines items of interest - the Ipswich Emergency System, In-theatre training certification, various Papers presented at Conferences and so on.

CONTENTS - PART ONE: 8

ILLUSTRATIONS.

THE FORMATIVE YEARS:

The Formation and growth of the Ambulance Service:

i. In Europe. ii. In Queensland – CATB; QATBH; QATB; QAS.

The word Ambulance had its origin in a time of crisis and emergency, when man's need for assistance and compassion for his fellow man was at its greatest - this was in the 18th and 19th century battlefields of Europe and America, when the word 'Ambulance', derived from ambulare (L) to walk, was used to differentiate mobile medical aid from static Hospital aid.
Dominic Jean Larrey, born 1766, was Napoleon Bonaparte's Surgeon General and loyal friend, regarded as the father of the modern Ambulance Service.

Larrey conceived the idea for immediate battlefield medical care, so he proposed to Napoleon the plan for an Ambulance (mobile military hospital) organised to follow the advanced Guard in the same manner of the flying artillery.
In this he was successful, for he states, "I was authorised to construct a carriage which I called the 'Flying Ambulance.'

THE ORIGIN OF THE QATB, the Queensland Ambulance Service:
It was men from the Army Medical Corps who were the movers for what was to become the Queensland Ambulance Service.

Queensland was the first State in Australia in which a formal Ambulance Service was organised.
The catalyst was an incident which occurred at the Brisbane Agricultural Exhibition on the 11th August 1892 - "it was a beautiful day at the Brisbane Exhibition, the Ladies were dressed in their finest, some in crinolines, others with bustle and trains. Colourful parasols dotted the Members Stand.
The young men of the day, with an eye for the Ladies, paraded the paddock area in their linen shirts, fine breeches and polished riding boots.

All was excitement for the Maiden Hunters' Plate was about to be run - the wide eyed horses, held with tight rein by their jockeys, were prancing at the starting line - a hum of expectancy rose from the crowd as the Starter raised his arm, a green handkerchief in his hand.

Down dropped the Starter's arm, horses reared, THEY'RE AWAY - the horses sprang forward into the straight, jockeys as splashes of colour on their backs – horses jostling for a clear run - a ROAR from the crowd – ONE'S DOWN -
E. Echlin's horse had stumbled - jockey Echlin was thrown to the track and his horse rolled on him - WOMEN SCREAMED!
Some track assistants and bystanders ran to his aid, a four-wheeled Molly Brown cab was commandeered and driven at pace to the scene.
Dr. Sandford Jackson and Mr. Seymour of the Army Medical Corps saw the fall and moved to assist, but before they reached the casualty well intentioned bystanders had lifted Mr. Echlin, bundled him into the Cab without any treatment –

the Cab was driven off to the Hospital."

Due to the well meaning, emotional and untrained management of the patient, his injury of a simple fracture was damaged further to become a compound fracture - a most serious injury in those days from the risk of infection and death.

Mr. S. Warrian of the Army Medical Corps was so disgusted by this untrained action and the resultant further injury that he discussed the incident with other members of the Corps and it was decided to call a meeting on the 12th September 1892.

This set the date and agenda for the first formal meeting of the future Queensland Ambulance Service for the 22nd December, and held in the Courier Mail building."

At this formal meeting the question was raised as to whether the service would be controlled by the respected St. John Ambulance Service, but this was decided against, as, in the opinion of those present, "it did not provide a paid staff, nor would it allow the freedom of action necessary to build a Queensland Service."

Thus the C.A.T.B., the City Ambulance Transport Brigade was formed in 1892, to be the first formal Ambulance Service in Queensland and the first professional service, e.g. with fully paid staff.

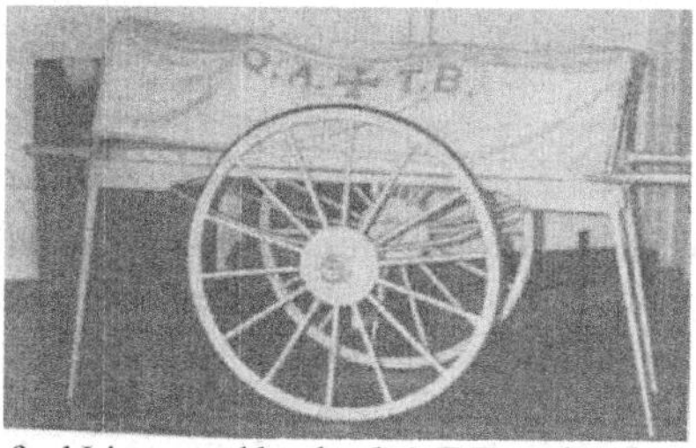

The Ashford Litter used by the C.A.T.B. and early Q.A.T.B.

Dr. J. Booth was the first Superintendent of the **C.A.T.B.**, with the following A.M.C. members as paid staff, E. Jack Captain, C. Elliott 1st Lieutenant, E. Rudd, 2nd Lieutenant and J.C. Harris Hon. secretary, S.C. Warrian Hon. Treasurer.

The staff was increased in January 1893 - an example of the wages being:- one pound per week for Officer in Charge Elliott, and 25 shillings per week for bearer W. Daniels.

The 1894 report of the City Ambulance Transport Brigade states that the Colonial Secretary granted the Brigade a donation of One Hundred pounds which was to receive the same rate of endowment as Hospitals and Charities.
The 1894 report provided statistics of:-

Accidents attended	357
Transports carried	344
False alarm calls	38
Total cases	739

Bearers travelled 1969.75 miles pushing the Ambulance Litter.
One of the objectives of the Brigade was: "The instruction of members of the elementary principles and practise of nursing and also of ventilation, especially in the sick room."
Members received lectures from local Doctors and from the Superintendent of the Brisbane Hospital, Dr. Sandford Jackson, and trained from textbooks of the Australian Medical Corps.

In 1895 the new service was recognised by the Government granting it financial support of a subsidy of one pound for every pound raised.

Towards the close of 1895, Mr. S. Warrian with K. Page and W. Mac Dermott, lead the establishment of the Ambulance service in New South Wales with the Civil Ambulance and Transport Brigade.
The State of Victoria had a limited service of litters used by the Police force until 1896 when the Fire Brigade manned the service till 1907. The service was conducted by a private contractor from 1907.

Even in 1901 the fledgling service in Queensland had its detractors, the following criticism recorded as from a member of the British Medical Association:

Press Report: OUSTED PROFESSION:
"There has of late arisen a body of men who have completely ousted the Medical practitioners in and around Brisbane from attending cases of accident or emergency. Originally started by two or three, enthusiastic as ambulance bearers solely, they soon claimed the right to administer first-aid in the case of accident in the absence of Medical men, and never think of obtaining Medical assistance for any case they are called to, but act together on their own responsibility, and even attend people who go to the Ambulance depot and in some cases have been known to attend people in their own homes.
This so called Ambulance Brigade has succeeded in obtaining the confidence of the public that, in the case of accident nowadays, no one ever thinks of sending for a Medical man, but the Ambulance Brigade is rung up, and they gallop along the street in a dog-cart painted yellow and drawn by a grey pony, the driver blowing lustily at a whistle to draw the attention of the people in the street as they pass."

That was an individual opinion in 1901, and we have heard more contemporary opinion in similar vein over succeeding years of the 20th century.

Prior to 1912 Tasmanian records show the establishment of horse drawn vehicles.

The Australian Capital Territory was run by the Fire Brigade from its inception in 1925 to 1955, after which it was run by the Canberra Hospital Board, and in 1968 the Health Services Branch of the Commonwealth Department became responsible for the service.

In Western Australia the Fire Brigade was responsible for calls to assist the injured until 1922 when the St. John Ambulance Association conducted the State Ambulance Service.

The South Australian service consisted of eight separate suburban enterprises in Adelaide with another eight independent country services operating until 1950 when a Royal Commission recommended that the Ambulance Service be restructured into a State system conducted by the St. John Ambulance Council.

The service in those early days was staffed by officers dedicated to providing the best patient care available, often purchasing equipment from their own funds, and always working to improve procedures and treatments.

The standard of the early Queensland service can be gauged by the inquiry from the London journal 'First Aid' which asked of the C.A.T.B.:-
"We learn with great interest that you have a unique installation of Ambulance service in your city, much in advance of what we possess here.
We would much esteem it if you can give us information respecting your Corps, and also lend us any illustrations or blocks of your Litter-sulky and other appliances.
We shall be pleased to record the work you are doing."

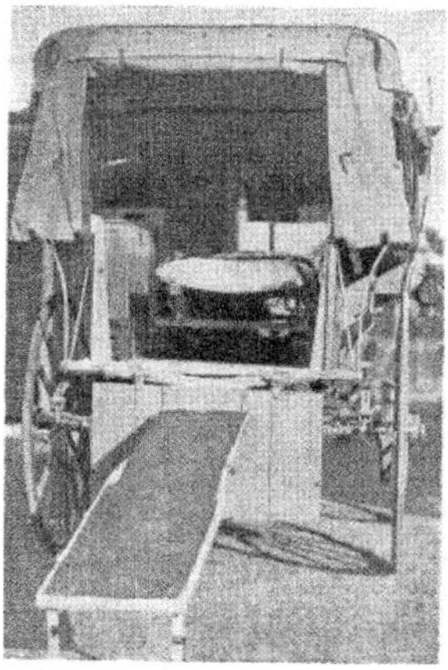

Interior and back view of first ambulance wagon.

Exterior and back view of the first Ambulance Wagon

Since that time many changes have taken place in the Ambulance service, but the ideals of the dedicated officer have remained constant, that of the care and welfare of the patient coming before self, and the ever striving to gain greater knowledge so that even better treatment might be achieved for the benefit of the patient.

This unique service spread further afield with Centres established at Townsville, Charters Towers, Rockhampton, Warwick and Ipswich.
Some affiliated with the C.A.T.B. and some independent.

In 1902 a change in the authority of the service was required and the Q.A.T.B.H. (Queensland Ambulance Transport Brigade Hospital) was established under the Hospitals Act, allowing autonomy to each Centre Committee to operate under the amended "Rules" and a State Executive to provide co-ordination between all Committees and to allow distribution of Government subsidies.

Toowoomba opened in 1902,
Mackay in 1903,
Ravenswood in 1903,
Cairns in 1904,
Ipswich in 1906,
Bundaberg in 1907.

In 1910 Rules were framed for the Q.A.T.B.H., and amended in 1919.

THE FRONTIER of the SERVICE – north Queensland

The officers and their families of this infant service suffered 'frontier' style hardships when they were establishing a new Centre and providing a service to the community, as can be demonstrated from records of the Wowan sub-centre.

"Mr. W.G. Nash was the first Officer-in-charge of the Wowan sub-centre of the Q.A.T.B.H. Mt. Morgan, and in October 1917 took up residence with his wife and family in a tent, and a lean-to with a galvanised roof for cooking.
The Ambulance wagon and horse were housed in a shed at the back of the tent."
This humpy like structure served for 12 months until a two story wooden building was constructed. This was dedication of the highest.

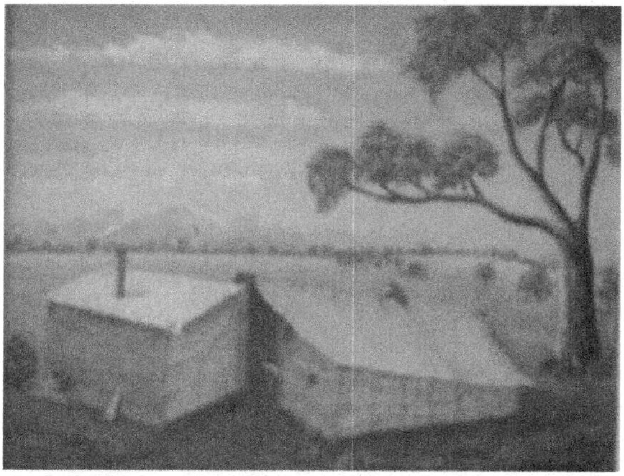
Artists illustration from a Newspaper extract of the time.
Temporary Gatton sub-centre of QATB Mt. Morgan

"In 1918 flood water was a foot deep in the tent, and in the same year the pneumonia influenza epidemic swept through the district, and Mrs. Nash was placed in charge of a temporary holding Hospital at the public hall, where patients were nursed until they could be transported to Mt. Morgan hospital 32 miles away."
This transport was on a stretcher loaded into the Ambulance wagon pulled by the traditional 'gray' horse.

The Ambulance Bearer drove the horse and wagon to the half-way point where the railway line crossed the Wowan - Mt. Morgan road.
This was where patients were transferred into the Mt. Morgan Ambulance, as prearranged by an earlier manual telephone call.

AMBULANCE SERVICE IN THE SOUTH JOHNSTONE DISTRICT.

A new Sugar Mill was established at South Johnstone in 1915 and with further land clearing for farming there was an increase of cases attended by the QATBH Cairns sub centre at Innisfail.

This larger production of cut sugar cane in the Japoon Valley area necessitated the construction of Cane Tramlines from the Valley back to the South Johnstone Sugar Mill.
The increased workforce on the farms made greater demands on the Ambulance service resulting in the QATBH Cairns Committee appointing Station Officer Henry Anderson to Japoon Valley, later assisted by Honorary Officer John Hendry in administering to workmen and farm families along the Japoon and Liverpool Creek tramlines. ref. "History of the Qld Ambulance"

In 1917 a sub-centre was built on Mill land at South Johnstone and in 1919 a Public meeting resolved "that a Centre of the QATB be established at South Johnstone." The plant consisted of a rail ambulance and stretchers.

Fred Gillam served at the QATBH south Johnstone in around 1930 under Superintendant W.J. (Bill) McConachie and in 1973 as a 'part time' Collector at Gatton Centre in 1973 at age 73. He recalled how the Ambulance Centre operated from Mill land and that there were only rough tracks or no road at all to the numerous cane farms and residences.

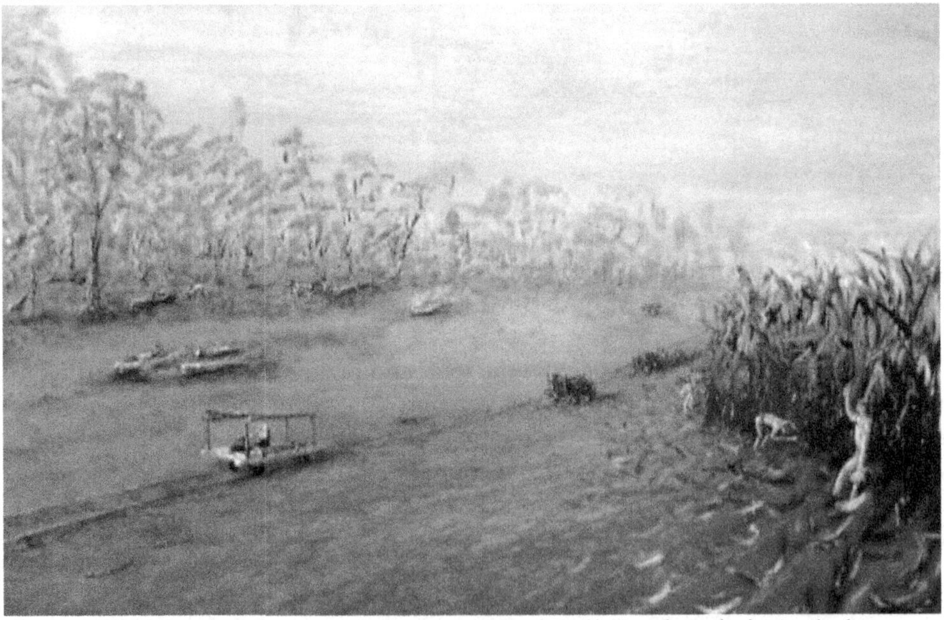

The QATBH South Johnstone had a motorised Rail Quad as their Ambulance Transport vehicle.
It had a hood and canvas blinds for protection. It carried a wood framed canvas stretcher attached to the tray of the railway Quad.
This serviced the farms in the District and was the Ambulance Vehicle to attend emergencies from snake bite, severe wounds/amputations from razor sharp cane knives, victims of Loco derailments, and the average domestic accidents and illnesses.

The Sugar Mill tram lines were the lifeline for the farm families as the excessive rainfall changing the red soil tracks to muddy quagmires, so farmers and their families used the Mill 'loco bus' via the cane loco tram lines as their means of communication with the Mill and the Township.

The painting was drawn from the stories told to me by Fred and from my memories of the clearing of virgin forests with axe, horse snigging of logs, and of early cane cutters and farming in the Cairns and Innisfail districts.

So much for 'the old days.'

The dedication and enthusiasm of the Bearer in those early days was exactly similar to that of our dedicated officers of today, for in my appointments to various centres throughout Queensland, I have found text books of a very high standard for their day, now dusty and put away.

Books ranging from Gray's Anatomy 1880 - Medicology by Joseph Richardson Professor of Hygiene, University of Pennsylvania 1908 edition - Manual of Splints and Appliances reproduced by permission of the United States Army, issued by the British Red Cross society 1917- Warwick and Tunstall's First Aid to the Injured and Sick, an Advanced Ambulance Handbook and -
Murrell's "What to do in cases of Poisoning."

The Treatment administered for a Wasp Sting in the early part of this century:-
Treatment:- 1. Make the patient lie down and give stimulants freely. Brandy, whisky and champagne are useful. If swallowing impossible, inject with an enema apparatus, into the rectum.

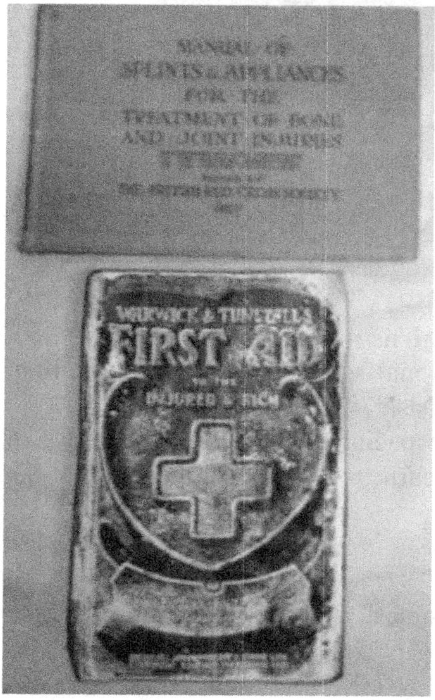

Thankfully treatments have improved and changed over the years:-
On the front shelf were copies of Sears, Anatomy and Physiology for Nurses;
Miller and Keane Encyclopaedia and Dictionary of Medicine and Nursing etc.

EARLY TREATMENTS AND APPLICATIONS.

World War I provided a number of 'discoveries' as to treatments and techniques which were lauded as the most modern and were made available in publications such as the "Manual of Splints and Appliances reproduced by permission of the United States Army," issued by the British Red Cross society 1917

It is understandable that these treatments administered to patients in those early days are looked upon as 'primitive' today, but in those times of a progressive Ambulance service, they were state of the art.

The very early First Aid kits carried applications of:-
½ lb. Borasic acid.
½ lb. Borasic ointment.
5 ozs. Tincture of Arnica.
5 ozs. Smelling salts. Note: Sal. Volatile (Aromatic ammonium carbonate diluted with water was also given as a 'pick-me-up.'
Triangular bandages.
Various sized bandages.
Lint, cotton wool, tow.

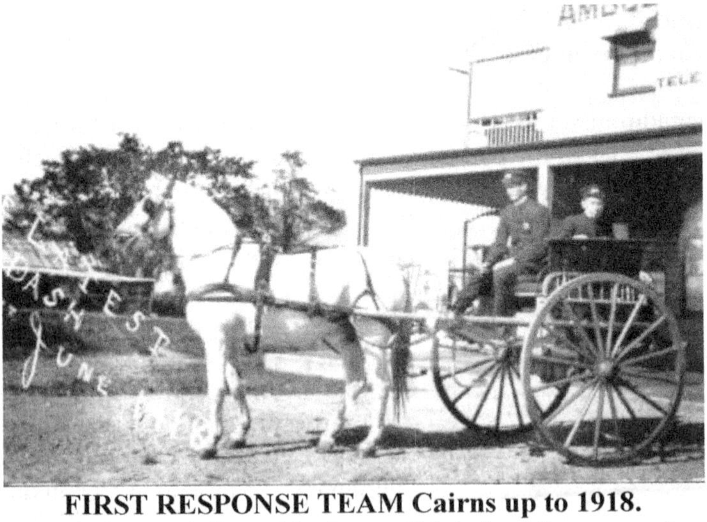

FIRST RESPONSE TEAM Cairns up to 1918.

The QATBH Ambulance Sulky with the traditional white pony chosen for their intelligence and spirit and appropriately named "Dash."
They were well cared for and stabled in stalls especially built for that purpose of immediate access having high racks holding the harness attached to the sulky at the rear of the stall.
There was a single slip rail at the front of the stall.

I well remember my father telling of the "white horses" of the Brigade.

When the telephone alarm bell sounded, the horse would move to the sliprail and stand under the harness. The Bearer would hurry out and release the harness sling so that the harness swung down onto the horses back.
As seen in the photo, the harness and sulky shafts was connected.

The other Bearer adjusted this and cinched the girth strap – the Bearer stepped up into the driver's seat, the second Bearer up behind him – the horse prancing ready to go. The Sliprail was dropped and the horse was away.

The magnificent spectacle of this spirited white horse, at a trot under tight rein, mane flying, tail up, the warning bell ringing, the Bearers braced upright and proud – what a sight they made.

Bearer Murphy with reins, Angus McDonald sitting – the Litter was generally pulled behind the Sulky to the accident/incident, and then the Bearers pushed the Litter with patient back to the Doctor or Hospital.

The motor vehicle was a contraption gaining acceptance, they were looked upon as being so dangerous as to warrant a person with a red flag to walk in front and for a bell to be rung to warn pedestrians of their approach.

Even so, the Brisbane Ambulance Committee were under pressure to attend accidents more quickly and in 1908 the Committee ordered a vehicle from the Canada Cycle Agency Limited for a four cylinder Clement Talbot Chassis. It duly arrived by boat in Brisbane and was immediately dispatched to Coach Builders to be fitted with a special ambulance body and was commissioned in May of 1909

Late 1918 the QATB Cairns installed their first Hupmobile Ambulance unit.

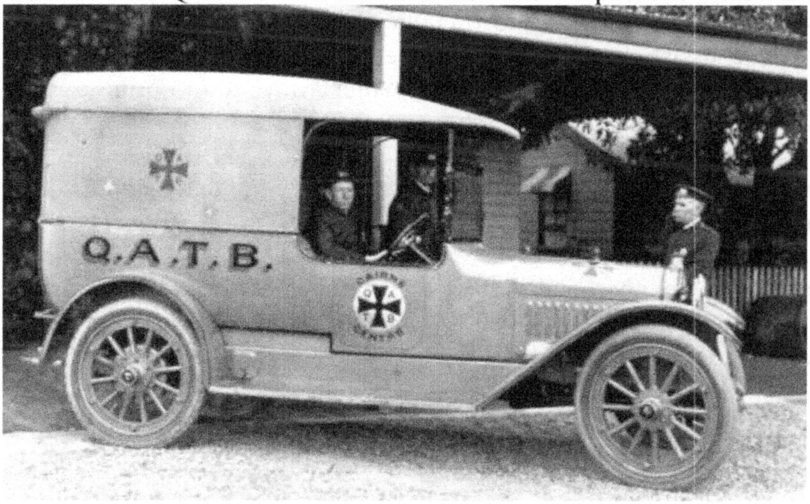

The first Driver Bearer in Cairns, Angus McDonald with Supt. Hogan.

ADVANCED FIRST-AID TREATMENTS - beginning of the 20th century.

Ambulance Driver Bearer of 1918, Angus McDonald explained specific treatments.

DEEP PUNCTURED WOUND from stepping on a nail or similar 'foreign object,' to combat the recognised danger from tetanus - other infection was secondary.
The area was cleaned with the antiseptic of the time, a weak solution of Condi's crystals, then a probe was dipped into caustic soda and inserted into the depth of the puncture, pushing the caustic soda to the bottom of the puncture – the intention was to cauterise the area to destroy any bacteria – it was rather painful, but it worked.

BURNS: Bicarbonate of Soda paste was applied to the burnt area, then a dressing and bandage

SNAKE BITE: a constrictive bandage applied above the bite to stop the flow of blood and poison past this point, and excise the bite site. Sucking of the wound and expectorating the saliva and 'poison' was also in vogue.

RED BACK SPIDER: incise the bite and cauterise with a red hot iron or apply strong nitric acid.
One wonders if the treatment might not have been worse than the cause, BUT, the death rate from untreated bites at that time was very high.

HOT FOMENTATION:
The recognised and accepted home and First-aid treatments of the early 20th century for various infections were Hot fomentation as appropriate for the specific condition - if there was inflammation or temperature, fight it with some form of heat.
Hot drinks (with lemon or medicinal additives), were administered, with the axiom "to sweat IT out"- one was never sure as to what the "IT" meant.
The reasoning was to assist the body to increase the circulation at the point of infection, to both flush the extraneous infectious matter away, and to bring oxygen and antibodies to fight the infection.

It was not until World War II that advances were made in the diagnosis and treatment of many diseases, ailments and internal injuries.

Advancement in research with the development of the identification of various infections and the medication to treat and cure were seen as miraculous as compared to the immediate past treatments and mortality.

TREATMENT FOR RESPIRATORY ARREST AND
ASTHMA.

A number of early resuscitation methods were trailed over a period. One of the earliest being the 'Barrel method' where the patient was draped face down over a large barrel and the barrel rolled back and forth causing some compression of the chest and stomach. This was to encourage drainage of the lungs and stomach and apply some pressure to the chest.

A resuscitation method still valued in the late 1950s was the Sylvester method:
As the adjacent diagram shows, the danger of airway obstruction from the tongue was appreciated and the instruction was for, "an assistant must catch hold of the patient's tongue with a handkerchief, draw it forward as far as possible and hold it in this position."

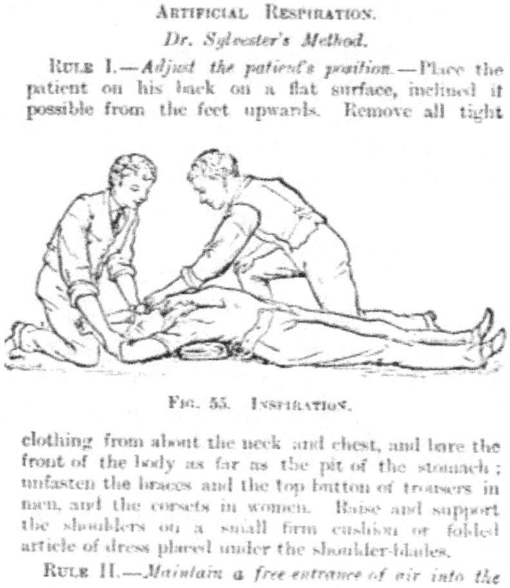
ARTIFICIAL RESPIRATION.

Dr. Sylvester's Method.

RULE I.—*Adjust the patient's position.*—Place the patient on his back on a flat surface, inclined if possible from the feet upwards. Remove all tight clothing from about the neck and chest, and bare the front of the body as far as the pit of the stomach; unfasten the braces and the top button of trousers in men, and the corsets in women. Raise and support the shoulders on a small firm cushion or folded article of dress placed under the shoulder-blades.

FIG. 55. INSPIRATION.

RULE II.—*Maintain a free entrance of air into the*

The arms were grasped at the elbows and lifted onto the chest and pressed downwards to compress the thorax expelling air then released by drawing them above the head resulting in expansion of the chest – this was repeated at a set rate.

The Shafer method followed and as it was thought that carbon dioxide stimulated a breathing reflex, this was supported by the use of a carbon dioxide Inhaler on a compressed gas sparklet (as used for a drinks soda water bottle), as a stimulant for the patient to breathe.

In the 1950s the Holger Neilsen method came into use which was an improvement.

The E and J Resuscitation unit which operated on a positive and negative pressure from two 'C' size oxygen cylinders.

This was bulky and heavy and of undecided benefit. It was referred to by some medicos as "the clucking hen" from the noise of operation.
Suction apparatus of coiled tubing on the floor is noted at (15).

The E and J Resuscitation Unit demonstrated on following page:

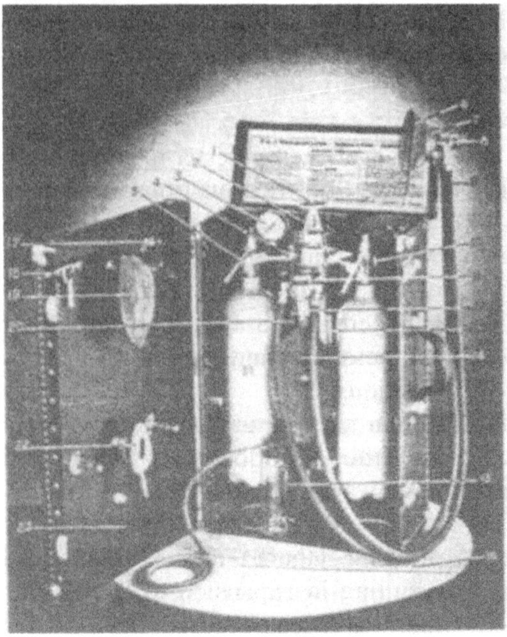

<u>The E.A.R. or expired air resuscitation</u> (mouth to mouth) method was introduced in the 1960s.
I was present at a demonstration of this revolutionary E.A.R. by then Dr. T. Brophy conducted in the First Aid station at the Cairns Wharf for First Aid officers.
The Doctor injected the patient with a respiratory paralysing drug whereby he ceased respirations.
The Doctor then applied E.A.R. until the drug wore off and the (now) patient breathed spontaneously.

Resuscitation techniques continued to progress over the years with the introduction of C.P.R. (Cardio Pulmonary Resuscitation), the application of which is still being refined in 2015.

Asthma was an unrecognised disease and was totally underestimated, being understood (at that time) to be a condition brought on by emotional circumstance similar to hysteria.
Thus the treatment was for the patient to have unrestricted clothing and access to fresh air.

Little else was done in the First Aid situation

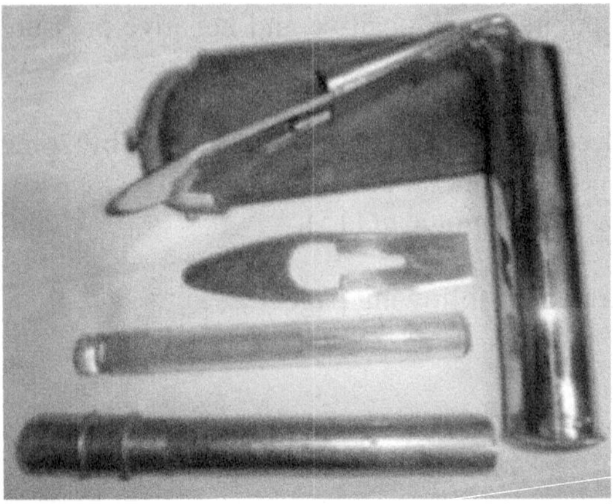

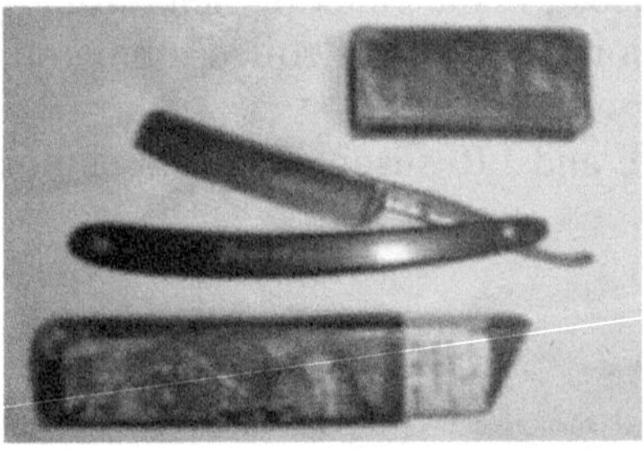

Early Laryngoscope and syringe (with container) used by the medical profession.

EDUCATION 1940 IN NORTH QUEENSLAND – THE FRONTIER.

This next segment is simply an aside to demonstrate that in those days, before civil libertarianism, anti discrimination, teen rights and of 'being precious,' there was a dark side whereby one might be injured from personalised attack.

Yes, the childhood protection mantra against "name calling," of, *"sticks and stones may break my bones but names will never hurt me,"* did not meet every obstacle a teenager might be called to face at that time in life - it was like this:-

Scholarship was [then] a very important event in the life of a young person for it was the time when you were tested as to whether or not you attained entry to the High School, the secondary school system, and today was THE DAY for me.

As I left home I saw Mr. Fitchett, an ex High School Industrial subject teacher, and a World War 1 servicemen who suffered from being gassed in that war, (each breath he took was an effort, he would take a great gasp of air and the veins in his neck would distend), he was six foot six in height, a fearsome vision.
As I walked past I raised my hat and said, "good morning Mr. Fitchett," he stopped me with the statement, "scholarship exams today Malcolm!" to which I replied, "yes Mr. Fitchett."

He fixed me with his severe stare, raised his foot and said, "see that, it's a size 13, and if you don't pass your scholarship you'll get it fair up your behind !" to which I replied, as a young lad in those days would, "yes, Mr. Fitchett," and walked on.
Needless to say I did pass my Scholarship but I don't think it was due to that implied threat.

Today this would be looked upon (by some) as potential injury and child abuse, but it was the style of interest and influence given by neighbours and men to any and all young people in those days.

It was the era when books gave the messages of :- 'protect your loved ones, even to sacrificing your own life,' and 'always go the extra inch or yard,' and to 'do your best for your country,' and 'honesty is the best policy,' and 'respect your elders,' all those things that made up a 'code of living' – a learning of wisdom.

Yes, I gained my 'Scholarship' and went on to attend at the Cairns High and Technical College for two years studying eight subjects, English, mathematics, geometry, algebra, chemistry, physics, Industrial1 Trade Drawing and Industrial 2 Woodwork.
I gained the Junior Public Certificate.
In the first few days at 'High School,' we were repeatedly informed that we were now 'students' in secondary education as opposed to previously being 'pupils' in the primary grades, the difference being that teachers were there to show and

demonstrate new knowledge, but *we were now expected to be responsible for our own study and efforts,* whereas in Primary education we were 'taught.'

This was nowhere more aptly demonstrated than in the Chemistry classes where Mr.[cyclone] Clarkson ruled. Teenagers did not necessarily feel that the gaining of knowledge was serious, BUT if you were one of Mr. Clarkson's students, YOU HAD BETTER BELIEVE IT.

Cyclone Clarkson was of slim build, not tall, but full of energy.
He earned his name from his actions and manner. He spoke in quick, crisp, clear sentences, and always walked at a fast pace; one would think that there was never enough time in the day for him.

He had a unique way of imprinting a lesson on the minds of students – he used voice intonation, visual example, shock moments, blackboard equations, gestures – *plus the odd humorous aside,* all to direct and keep attention on the subject – an example for future leaders and lecturers to note.

Our first chemistry lesson started with 'Cyclone' giving a demonstration at the front bench and informing us that:- "this was a mortar and this a pestle, [scoop of sulphur], and they were used, [scoop of charcoal], to grind and to mix carefully,[scoop of potassium nitrate], NEVER to bash or pound, [tapping the pestle against the rim of the mortar, another stir], because,[pours a small mound of the mixture onto a metal plate], you don't know, [picks up a hammer], what may result." **BANG** as he struck the powder with the hammer, and a cloud of smoke rose to the ceiling - we near died – WE WERE IMPRESSED.

This was followed with him talking about solutions and gases, again listing the equipment:- " this is a gas chamber,[the sealed chamber with glass sides and a sealed vent for gaseous experiments], this is a bell jar", and so on.
Whilst he was talking, he took hydrochloric acid and sodium chlorite, so that a sinister plume of dirty green gas was generated within the gas chamber, 'cyclone' then informed us that this was chlorine gas, used in the 1st. World War and capable of virtually dissolving your lungs if breathed in - he then let a minuscule whiff of gas to escape into the room,

WE SMELT IT and, as he intended, WE NEVER FORGOT IT - in the first minutes of his very first lesson 'cyclone' had established a safety barrier in the use of chemicals and of equipment that the class would always remember and obey.
It was he who endeavoured to teach us to think for ourselves, to put aside the 'learn by rote' method that had been so necessary to the amassing of certain knowledge and theorems - but it was again in his indubitable style.
All students had passed their Scholarship examinations to attain entry to Secondary education, as this was a major examination in regards to their future in life, all had studied hard to ensure they passed.

'Cyclone' asked a question, and the student answered off pat, [simply rattled off the answer without having to think, as learned from the text book], - to the amazement of the student, [whose answer was correct], 'Cyclone' would yell from the front of the class, "*like a sausage machine, like a sausage machine, turn the handle and out it comes, turn the handle and out it comes,*" he would then give the example of how the student should think first and then provide an answer in their own words.

After a few months the class progressed to carrying out chemical experiments in the laboratory, some of which had somewhat complicated and expensive equipment, so one can imagine the care with which the students worked - the unthinkable - the sound of a piece of equipment striking the floor - "*what was that* ?" came the staccato question from somewhere in the room.
A tremulous voice answered, "*it fell Sir*."
The incredulous reply, "*it fell ! it fell! an inanimate object moved ? for every reaction there must be a corresponding action - a force must be applied for any action to take place*," etc.

So, no matter what took place there was always a scientific theorem quoted or lesson given, we might not have appreciated the manner, but we never forgot the lesson.
SOMEWHAT DIFFERENT TO SCIENCE CLASSES IN 2016.
The science subjects of chemistry and physics provided essential basic knowledge to understand anatomy, physiology and the basic principles of medicine in later years.

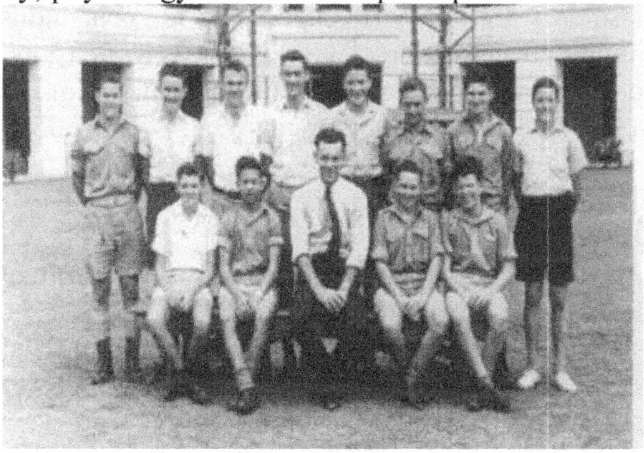

Students of the Industrial subjects.
David Lyle; Bill Sexton; George Lawrence; Graham Golightly; Don Mackenzie; Billie Eddie; Christianson. [front] Peter Loveland; Ronnie Tong; Dave Dunstan; Don Eddleston; Malcolm McDonald

The two years at the Cairns High and Technical College soon passed and the final examinations took place over a period of one week - then came the wait for the results to be printed in the local and State papers - page 8, where ? WHERE? - McDonald, M.C, yes, yes, A's, B's and a couple of C's, good enough, passed the lot.

What next ?

I was the sixth child and one went to work.
There was no thought of not working in 1950, everyone was looked upon to contribute, but WHAT?
I had no inclination as to what trade or profession I wished to follow, so it was up to fate to lend a hand.

Came the start of the new year and firms advertised for permanent staff and apprentices, so Dad and I had a discussion:-

Dad, " you have to look at your economic future," reply, "yes."
" you need a job that is secure, " reply, "yes."
" a trade is a sound base for the future," reply, "yes."
" a government department gives job security," reply, "yes."

Well that was decided. An apprenticeship in a Government Department and with a Junior pass I was sure of a position.
The positions advertised were mainly for the Railway, and of those listed I chose the clean and diverse trade of Car Trimmer in the Cairns Railway Workshops - I was a 'Little Trimmer.'

I signed up for 5 years as an indentured apprentice, and when you read the fine print, your life was not your own anymore.
Teachers and Tradesmen were not only responsible for your industrial training but also for your rectitude and could direct you as far as your (good) behaviour was concerned, and you were liable for certain punishment if you misbehaved or did not obey direction, you had signed your freedom away.

This was the start of my (later) chosen career.

The only interruption allowed to my Apprenticeship was official, in 1952 I was 'called up' for National Service.

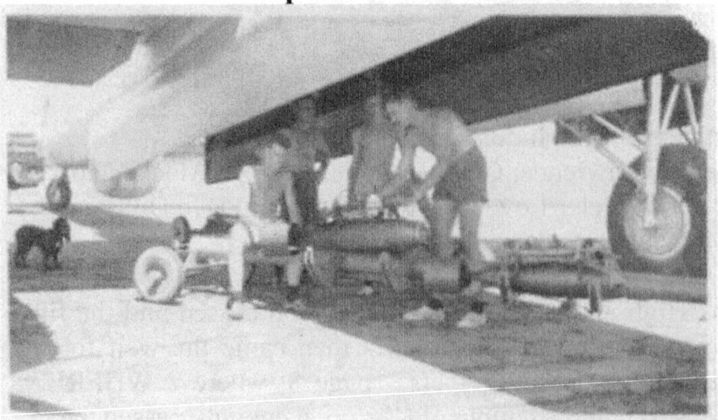

ACR Malcolm McDonald, armament fitter 10 (OP) Squadron Garbutt.

INTRODUCTION TO THE AMBULANCE FRATERNITY.

I may have had something of an introduction to the Ambulance Service from my Father serving in the QATBH thirty-one years before, but inadvertently my entry into an Apprenticeship in the Railway Department introduced me to my calling, the vocation I was to embrace wholeheartedly as my professional career.

IPSWICH - the Home of Queensland Railway Ambulance Corps.

The last year of my apprenticeship was spent at the Ipswich Railway Workshops so that I experienced the complete requirements of my trade.
In the Trimming shop I worked under different tradesmen gaining experience in specific sections of the trade.
One tradesman was Alf Grieves who cut the expensive chrome leather hides to size for seats, sleeper bunks and special furniture.
This allowed him to be interrupted at any time to carry out his special duties.

It was here that I was introduced in 1954 into the QRAC (Queensland Railway Ambulance Corp) through Alf who was a First Aid Attendant for the Ipswich Railway Workshops from his station in the Trimming Shop.
There were other Fist Aid stations but injured tradesmen would bypass those to come to Alf for attention.

During this time I attended the First Aid course at the Queensland Railway Ambulance Corps classes during my lunch hour and found them most informative and interesting; *I studied hard so as not to disgrace myself* and gained a high pass.

This drew the attention of the manager of the Railway Ambulance Competition team who asked me to come along to the practise sessions.

The Competition practise sessions consisted of scenarios of an accident scene with an injured patient, and the competitor entered the room and had to examine and treat the patient asking the appropriate questions to identify the patient's condition and injuries to allow for a diagnosis. These were answered by the marking adjudicator.

My problem was my peculiar sense of humour - the patients used for these practises did not have any mock 'simulated' injuries,[as they did in actual competitions and even those in 1953 were nothing like the 'make-up studio' injuries of later years], they only had a piece of sticking plaster on their arm or leg with 'wound' or 'fracture' written on it, so I could not take the exercise seriously and had to control myself from laughing at the unnatural pretence of it all.
This was to change later.

My high pass also gave me the opportunity to work with Alf in his capacity as the First-aid Attendant in the Trimming Shop.

He was a most particular, scientific and experienced Attendant.
He was so respected for his knowledge and expertise that Tradesmen from other sections of the Workshops would come to him for attention.

He worked from a glass fronted First-aid cabinet of instruments, dressings, solutions and ointments.
Yes, arnica for sprains, Tinct Benz co as a specific antiseptic, and smelling salts of Sal Volatile (Aromatic ammonium carbonate, diluted with water was also was given as a 'pick-me-up'), were solutions in use at that time.

The dressings, bandages and swabs were in separate marked jars and the cabinet was scrupulously clean and all instruments were scrubbed after use and placed in a disinfectant solution before return.
This example of cleanliness and attention to prevention of cross infection was a lesson that stayed with me.

Some instruments were especially made to Alf's design by the Blacksmiths and plated by the Nickel-platers to assist in his no-touch technique.

In 1954 the Ipswich Workshops had a complement of 4000 people working in the trades of blacksmith; boilermaker; fitter and turner; carriage builder; painter; car trimmer; welder; electrician; pattern maker and moulder as well as engine driver and shunter.
All type of light and heavy machinery was in use providing ample opportunity for accidents to occur.

The majority of injuries were cuts, abrasions, bruises and strains, foreign bodies to hands and eyes and eye injury from welders flash.
There were lesser numbers of fractured arm and collar bone and the odd fractured leg, plus an heart attack now and then – all in all a most instructional variety of injuries.
The treatment of small cuts at the eyebrow and small deep abrasions were Alf's speciality and was the same as used for Boxers in the ring – i.e. the wound was carefully cleaned with swab and antiseptic, and then cleaned again and again to ensure any possible infective material was removed.
A sterile swab was pressed over the wound to align the edges, control bleeding and to maintain asepsis.

A solution of Tinct Benz co was painted over the wound immediately followed by a fine tease of cotton wool, further Benz co, more wool, Benz co etc until a compact thin dressing of cottonwool and Benz co sealed the wound from any external agents and bleeding was controlled.
This dressing dried very quickly as it was being applied and gave a tough protection that would resist water and any pollution from the working environment – the tincture of Benz co also "stung like hell" at first requiring the clenching of teeth to

stifle a groan from pain.
This type of dressing allowed the tradesmen to continue in their work environment.

Shortly after this, Alf wanted to take some of his holidays and asked me if I would do his job of First-aid Attendant as I had served a type of 'apprenticeship' with him. I was somewhat reticent but after some encouragement from Alf I agreed.

The day before Alf left he once again ran through the duties of the First-aid Attendant with me.
I said that I felt a bit concerned due to my lack of experience, "don't worry Malcolm, we all have to start somewhere, the day I started the band-saw broke and wrapped itself around the wood machinist, it was a bit of a job patching him up, blood everywhere."

With that gem of reassurance to me Alf left and went on his holidays.

The few weeks did pass without any major problems, just the average cuts, foreign bodies, burns and sprains, although I almost, yes almost, had a real case:-
The workshop's whistle blew to restart work after the morning smoko break and about ten minutes later I heard a commotion:

" **first-aider!, FIRST-AIDER! needed at the gantry crane !**"

I grabbed my first-aid kit and hurried to the caller and followed him to the overhead gantry crane which carried all the timber into and out of the wood machine shop.
A group were gathered at the base of the gantry looking up at the crane-operator's cabin 25 feet up.

I could see the operator sitting in his seat with his head back against the wall, there was no movement.

I climbed up the vertical steps, reached the cabin and looked inside.
The operator had seemingly gone to sleep and had fallen backwards in his seat so that the back of his head touched the wall.

The problem was that the wall had the junctions and terminal posts of the electric power cables into the cabin with the wiring for the controls of the electric motors of the crane - ***they were bare*** - not covered with insulation – it was a most dangerous situation.
The accident had occurred at least 20 minutes ago - there was nothing to be done.

I backed down the ladder, reported to the Shop foremen and ordered all power to be cut off from the crane. The Police were called.

In 1954 the Government was free of any Regulations for Government owned and run workshops etc, and there were no Regulations covering Workplace Health and Safety.

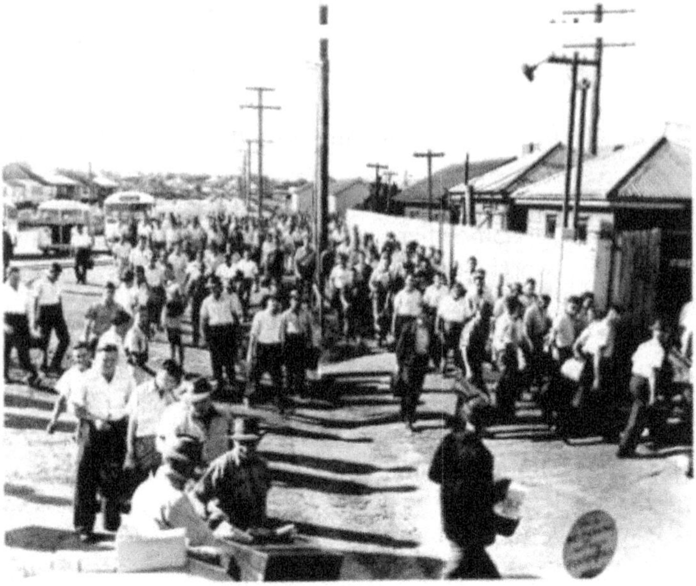

Ipswich Railway Workshop staff 1954-5.

RUN FOR IT –
even this unlikely event provided practical Ambulance experience.

The workforce in the Ipswich Railway workshops was 4000 strong, made up of tradesmen from numerous trades plus skilled and unskilled assistants; these men came from all walks of life and had diverse interests so that one would find coaches, trainers, judges, starters, athletes of all the amateur sports.

In November of 1954 a couple of apprentices asked me, "can you run ?"

I wondered what this was all about, so replied, " a bit."

"What's your time for the 100 ?"

Time for a 100 yards !! In the north we *simply ran,* we didn't worry about *the time* it took, only who won and who came second, so I had to reply,
"I don't know my time for 100, but I can run a bit."

A group of apprentices then organised a 100 yards sprint championship.
Trimmers made numbered lane patches for the runners, Metal Turners had the large concrete area cleared of carriage wheels and axles - this area was over 100 yards long and about 50 yards wide.
Starters, Judges and timekeepers from Sports Clubs came from the Carriage shop, Metal shop and the Trimming shop.
Painters marked out the lanes and Linkmen measured the distance.

The whistle blew for the one hour lunch break, the big day had finally arrived, there were six lanes and there were to be a number of heats, with the first and second placed to run in the final. I was pretty nervous,
(1) Because I did not know the capabilities of the other runners, but they did.
(2) Because I was 'from the North' and had to keep the 'honour' of the 'northerners,' but could I?

It was a hot summer day, I pretended to fool around but in reality I was trying to limber myself up without appearing to do so *and yet keep myself calm and control my adrenaline flow, so that I could use it when I needed it for* a fast start.

My heat lined up, each of us with our lane number, some with sandshoes, no running shoes, [I didn't own a pair anyway], only bare feet.
"On your mark - are you set" - BANG went the starter's gun - we were off, the 100 yards of concrete stretched before us.

I concentrated on reaching the finishing line first, three quarters down the track I stumbled on a break in the concrete, but recovered to finish in front. As I slowed I felt this burning to my feet, then strong pain when I stopped.

I sat down and Alf Grieves [the First-aid attendant] checked my feet, I had two patches of skin off the sole of my foot, we thought it must have occurred when I stumbled on the crack in the rough concrete.

Well the Finals had to be put off until my foot had healed.

Alf cleaned the raw area of any sand, then using 'no touch technique' cleaned it again and again with antiseptic, dried it with a sterile swab, then dressed it with Tinct Benz co and cotton wool,[the same application used for the cut above a boxers eye from a blow in a match], but did it sting!! It stung right through my body.
It must be noted that Alf was so fastidious that he had special instruments made and Nicol-plated to assist in asepsis and in providing a high standard of treatment from his First-aid station – he was a leader in his field.

So a couple of weeks later we lined up again, but this time it was only the winners and it was for the Championship.

BANG, and we were off, *'GO, you must not be beaten,'* I told myself, I concentrated on the finish line - through, and first.

I slowed down, and the burning, the pain, it was worse than before, I hopped to a stop and sat down on the hot concrete.

I looked at my feet, both feet had been injured, there were patches of raw flesh to the balls of both feet, it had not been the stumble which had caused my injury in the first heat.
What had occurred was that the concrete was so hot that the [toughened], skin on my feet had softened, and then the friction of my running had caused the sole to blister, then the blister had lifted and the skin torn off.

Well I had won, but at a price - later I found I had officially run the 100 yards in 11.4 seconds, which was not too bad for bare feet, the rough track and the hot conditions.
Alf Grieves dressed both feet this time and I nearly fainted from the pain of the application, but he was so expert at his craft that I was still able to do my daily swimming training for my Royal Lifesaving Bronze Medallion, and the feet healed nicely.

The 'cup' for winning the championship was duly presented, it was a large china Railway Refreshment Room cup with "The 100 yards Trimmers Championship Cup of 1954" painted [by hand] across the front, a real honour and something to treasure.

Sportographs

(By T. G. N.)

Sprint . . .

Cairns apprentice, Malcolm Cameron McDonald, the rank outsider of the heats, won a 100yds. sprint at the workshops last week. The track, a concrete strip between the wheel shop and the mill, took heavy toll of the runners' bare feet, and an ambulance man was on the spot when the final was run to make immediate skin grafts. The championship resulted from a challenge by two lads in the trimmers' shop and developed into a field of eight. Two heats were run followed by the final a few days later when sore feet had recovered. Bruce Wilson was second in the final and Ron Oldmeadow third. The winner's time, 11.4secs., wasn't bad considering the running conditions. One of the slowest to begin, both in his heat and the final, Malcolm mowed the field down with a paralysing finishing burst. Could be a champion Rugby League winger in the making?

1955 – Ipswich Railway Workshops 100 yard sprint won by Cairns apprentice in 11.4 seconds.

This win gave me the introduction to play 'A' grade hockey for Eastern Suburbs team and to represent Ipswich in their Colts Representative team in 1955.

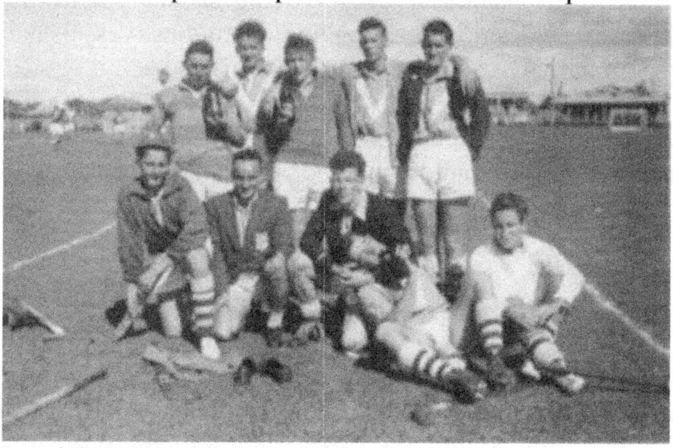

Ipswich Colts at final of State Comps at Bundaberg - 1955

EARLY TRAINING :

After I returned to Cairns in 1955, I continued my studies and sat for the annual First-aid exams to qualify as a Railway Ambulance Corps attendant.
I was asked to be a member of the Cairns workshops competition team.
A 'team' was four First-aiders, one patient and a manager/coach, so I joined the team.

The Railway Ambulance conducted Regional and State Competitions each year, consisting of an Individual event and Teams events for Trauma, Improvised and for Transport.

A couple of months before the competitions we would train two evenings a week after work, administering to a patient with simulated injuries in an emergency scenario.

Col Wheat, a permanent Ambulance officer with the Q.A.T.B., would set all the scenarios and used 'artificial injuries' to make the accident realistic, and would adjudicate whenever he could.
This training required commitment and developed self discipline, for we took it seriously as a means of developing our skills and preparing us for any future emergency which could occur in the workshops or in the railway marshalling yards.

Our training stood us in good stead when called to respond to emergencies at different times.

One such actual emergency to which I was called was of a shunter whose boot had been caught between the edge of the moving wagon wheel and the railway line as he swung on a buffer to hook up the couplings of two wagons.

On examination I found the boot torn and loose. On removing same I found that 75% of the top of his left foot had been de-gloved exposing the tendons, vessels and bones of the foot as if in a dissection, there was very little haemorrhage.

I instructed that an Ambulance be called, applied dressings, padding and bandages. I then applied an L splint over padding to the ankle and foot and bandaged firmly to immobilise movement, (this was made of a tightly folded newspaper then bent into an L shape).
The QRAC 'team' then stretchered the patient across the railway tracks to the closest access road for the Ambulance.

I was involved in Competition work for five years and was fortunate to win Sate awards of 'The Minister for Transports Gold Medal' in 1957, The Thallon Gold Medal in 1958 and an 'Individual Gold Medal' in 1960, thanks to training from committed officers like Col Wheat.

The Team competitions were taken very seriously in regards to providing the correct treatment and patient management, it was most serious but it was all good fun, you worked as a team and assisted each other over any problems.

The Individual tests were a different matter.

As I had done well at my First aid theory and practical examinations, and won awards for theoretical test cases, I was expected to do well at the practical Individual operational scenarios.

In the Individual test, the competitors waited in a separate room away from the test arena and any other people, and waited to be called to compete, this could be a very trying time for competitors.
Mental pressure can be exacerbated by outside influences, but it is really self imposed - *it can be an asset or a destructive force.*

Your own self respect and the wish to put up a good effort to assess the patient's condition and to administer the correct treatment under the time constraint, with spectators checking every move, created the ideal situation of 'mental pressure' on the individual as might be experienced in an actual emergency situation.

I always felt this pressure as a heightening of nerves, but I learned to understand that it was an outpouring of adrenaline, and that I had to control this and to use it to my advantage.

I would first reassure myself that I had done my preparations, I had studied and trained, I had done what I could, so that was that - I would then concentrate on relaxing [as best I could] so as to conserve my energy and to hold the adrenaline until I needed it - I would rest back and study the other competitors and might even involve in some gamesmanship, such as creating an aura of confidence about myself and maybe giving them some doubts - *if you know how to do it you can better protect yourself from the same tactics.*

I would endeavour to keep my mind clear from the event ahead until called to compete - I now had 3 minutes to prepare - I now allowed the adrenaline to flow, I might even tremble a little or feel very calm but I was building to a pitch of concentration so that when the bell rang for me to enter the arena I was at full concentration, I was totally alert.
I did not see any spectators I only saw the test area, I saw every detail and analysed every bit of visual information - *thus I used this 'nervousness' to full advantage.*

But, when all is said and done, win lose or draw, it did not really matter, five minutes later no one cared, the main thing was to participate, to give it all you had, to enjoy the experience, *and if you learned something new or were able to improve on your ability, that was the benefit, that was the bonus.*

I learned to put aside what had just occurred, *because that was now past*, and look forward to the next event.
I would use this lesson in future years when I attended incidents involving serious injury, multiple trauma and the pressure from emotional family members.

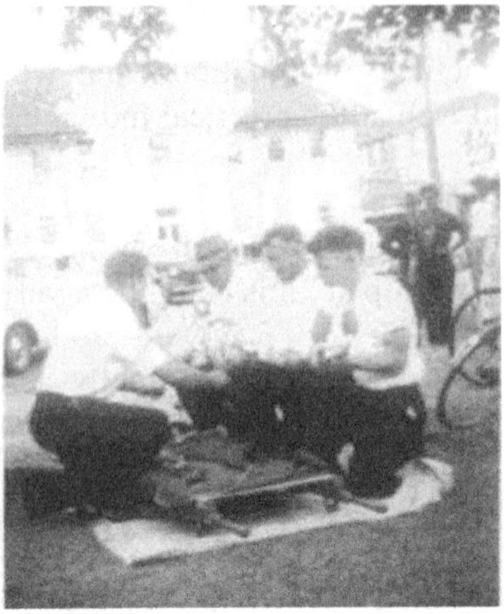
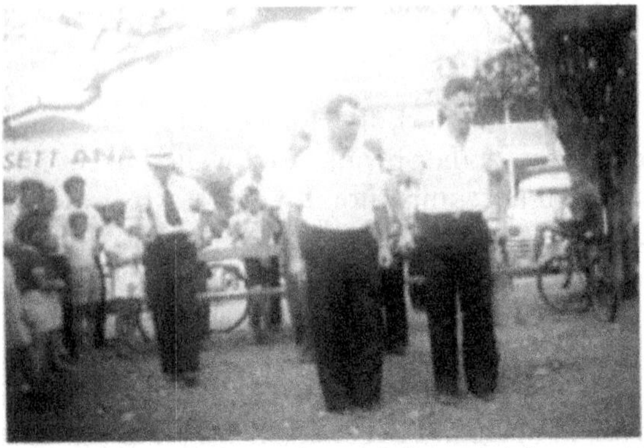

The Patient "Treat and Transport" (over obstacles) section of Competitions – 1957 Cairns Team.

I assisted with teaching First aid in 1959, attained my First aid Instructors Certificate in 1960 and instructed classes in Cairns until 1962.

There was no payment for lecturing classes.

I enjoyed lecturing to classes and received great satisfaction in imparting knowledge to others, especially when it could be of so much help to those in need.
Before each lecture session I made sure I had some visual effects to help the class understand 'why.'

When lecturing on fractures I would have prepared pieces of a sheep leg bone [soaked in weak acid solution for days to remove the calcium], to demonstrate the flexibility of bone in young people. I would also select a similar bone from a cooked shank to show the calcification and brittleness of older people's bones.

I worked on the principle that basic knowledge [of any subject] was of utmost importance if one was to know that subject well.

Basic knowledge was the foundation for further understanding of the subject, always be satisfied that you understand and learn the basic theorem or fact, concentrate on the start of any lecture, *if there was a chink in basic knowledge then there will be a large hole in the overall understanding of the subject.*

On the night of the Lecture I would show the flexible piece of bone demonstrating the early formation of bone in an infant --then I would show a green branch and bend this until it split demonstrating a greenstick fracture as in a child.

The hard bone was finally demonstrated as in an elderly person, explaining the change in the bone structure and fractures and supporting this by writing notes on the board.

Thus I would explain the structure of bone and demonstrate why fractures occur in the different age groups etc - all good fun.

In 1959 I joined the Cairns Q.A.T.B. as an Honorary Bearer.

THE Q.A.T.B. CAIRNS OPENS THE DOOR TO A NEW LIFE .

CAIRNS - THE AMBULANCE SERVICE, AS IT WAS.

I commenced my QATB honorary Ambulance service in 1959 at the QATB Cairns as an Honorary officer and continued in the Railway Ambulance Corp as a First-aid attendant and competed in QRAC Competitions

I soon found that this was my ‘calling’ in life and as my work ethic was to do your best at whatever you attempted I was soon committed to the delivery of emergency care to the best of my knowledge and ability.

Before the 70's all officers were called Bearers which was a continuation of the traditional 'stretcher bearer', when Bearers walked and carried the patient on a stretcher. Later the stretcher was placed on a two wheeled 'litter' which was pushed by Bearers.
In the First World War stretcher Bearers risked life and limb to carry the wounded out from the front line in the thick of the action, and earned great respect from all ranks.

In the 1950's a permanent 'Bearer' was a married man, [couldn't have a single chap treating females] tolerant, mature, sober, neat and of clean habits, the holder of First-aid and Home Nursing certificates and a Driver's license. He must have served as an Honorary Ambulance-bearer for a period of time and participated in fundraising activities.
A Home Hygiene Certificate was required later for the permanent service.

The Honorary service was the most important factor as far as choosing a good permanent officer, for an Honorary attended one night every week and worked on one week-end a month for no pay or reward, except for a uniform. You supplied your own ‘kit’ and instruments – the bandages and medications were supplied by the Centre.

He worked under the supervision of a permanent officer for any emergency case, but could be sent to carry out the transport of any patient who did not require specific treatment.

This Honorary service soon sorted out the dedicated people from those only attracted to the service for the drama and excitement, as duties consisted of assisting with sweeping and cleaning vehicles and rooms, cleaning and sterilising of dirty equipment, various mundane tasks,[even polishing all copper pipes and taps], and waiting, WAITING, for an emergency.

Honorary Bearers could attend night after night and not be called to any emergencies, and when they did go on a case you could be sure they got the 'heavy end' or the 'dirty job' as the junior.

This honorary position allowed the Service time to appraise new H/Bearers and for the bearer to learn just what the service entailed, thus the person could leave if they found the job not to their expectations, or the Superintendent might suggest they were not suitable.

Some men joined the Q.A.T.B. as a community service, simply to help their fellows and gave their time freely for many years, others, like myself joined as a service to the community but after a time realised that this was our calling and we then applied for a permanent position at a Centre and invariably lost some money in wages, as most bearers were tradesman and the service paid just below a tradesman's wages.

NOTE: It can be seen that there were no Government policies on selection process, equal opportunity, discrimination or harassment etc. It may not have been the fairest or best method for choosing staff, but it certainly obtained the dedicated, those able to communicate and who had gained the respect of their peers, those who had few illusions of what the service was about.

Then the AMBULANCE SERVICE was a CHARITY and FUNDRAISING a necessity, a Bearer quickly learned the skills of communication and marketing – some better than others.

In the fifties the word FUNDRAISING covered a multitude of meanings, from Ambulance collectors calling on business firms for donations, or receiving pledges from cane growers to donate a halfpenny per ton of cane delivered to the mill.

Guilds and community groups were encouraged to conduct a fete, concert or event to raise finance on behalf of the Ambulance. Dances were conducted by Ambulance officers on their nights off, and the Ambulance Christmas Carnival ran annually for the three Friday and Saturday nights before Christmas.

This 'Carnival' had merry-go-round rides, fairy floss, lucky dips for the children, and various stalls, but the main attraction was the big Lucky Wheel [depending on whether you won or not] which had good quality prizes worthy of being given as Christmas presents.

The greatest attraction of the Lucky WHEEL were the large smoked legs of ham as a first prize. Legs of ham, then as now, were costly for the average family so the chance to win a large ham for 'two bob' was a temptation, and coupled with assisting a popular charity like the Ambulance, proved irresistible for most people.

You attended again the next night, and the following weekends until Christmas.

An unintended benefit from selling tickets was the training you received in human behaviour and in crowd management which are vitally important to any ambulance officer at a major incident or a home emergency.

No officers whether permanent or honorary were paid, nor were the many other helpers who assisted in these major fundraising activities.

This was looked upon as community service, and a highly respected one at that.

LIFE IN THE FAST LANE - A little knowledge can cause concern.

Life is what you make it, full of experiences, some ordinary, some uplifting, some rewarding, and some simply exciting – all rich grist to the mill of understanding human nature which was to be of great value in my future.

The motorcycle was the symbol of the man in the fast lane, and to be a Scramble Rider and Trick Motorcyclist was seen by some, as being at the top – to me, it was just great fun.
The leather clad figure in crash helmet and riding boots crouched over the motorcycle. He was a part of this roaring machine as it raced over the T.T. Course on the now dry, tidal mud flats at Smith's creek, Cairns in the late 50's.

His concentration was total - gauging the distance to the sweeping corner approaching at speed, he kept the throttle open to the ultimate second before throttling back and opening up with a racing change down through the gears to throw the machine in a power slide into the left hand corner, smell of heat, dust and oil in the air.
Adrenaline was high as he controlled the slide, left leg dragging, rear wheel sliding at a right angle to the line of travel, power on to hold the slide, front wheel pointed to bring this hot, roaring, hundredweight of machinery out of the slide back upright and into the back strait.

He had walked the track three times before the racing started so that he knew the layout and angles for cornering and had ridden practise laps to calculate the best line for the greatest speed through the corners.

He was now committed, on line, at speed, into this corner – WHAT! - a stray mongrel dog on the track - a lift and sway of the body to slide around the animal - power kept on to control the machine – it was sliding out wide, but all's well - Noooo, a deep wheel rut in the track - front wheel sinks - props - the machine and rider somersault into the air and into the mangrove trees.

The rider lay dazed, but his Ambulance training kicked in. He mentally did a primary assessment to check that all systems are GO - yes conscious - yes CAN move head, arms and legs - yes CAN stand - good I'm O'K - stands and takes a step to walk away, but his right leg is limping –

IT'S SHORTER THAN THE LEFT LEG-
SSSssugar I've FRACTURED ME FEMUR !!

He sat down to do a secondary assessment -- AH! she's jake! the crash simply ripped off the full sole and heel of the heavy riding boot, reducing the overall length of the right leg by one and a half to two inches – a concern for anyone with First-aid knowledge.

He walked nonchalantly off the track and over to his future wife, to show he's safe [and tough as nails, of course], but a great training experience.

What a great week-end it's been, hockey fixtures yesterday, (we won naturally),took my Sunday school class of 14 year olds this morning, a couple of good races after lunch (before the crash and splitting the crash helmet), later a barbecue with the club, and taking my girl, [Val], home - what a life.

So, the primary assessment must be followed by a methodical secondary assessment to make a correct diagnosis.

The Motorcycle era 1952 to 1960.

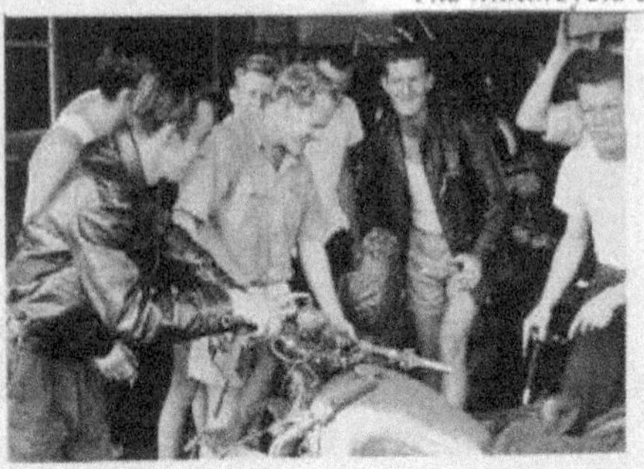

Pre race check.
Rusty Rees; Ernie Murphy; Malcolm McDonald and others in the old Llewellyn Motors workshop

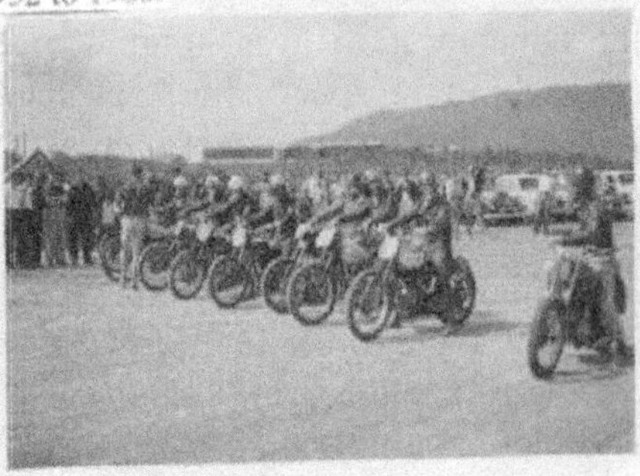

Race day – 1958
TT course at the Smith's Creek tidal flats.

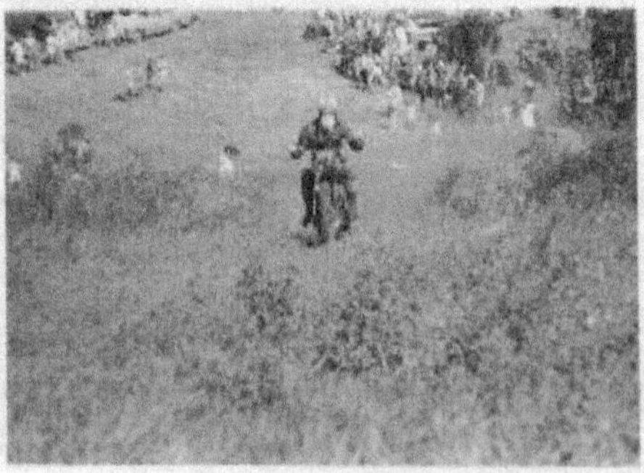

Freshwater Hillclimb- Cairns and District Motorcycle Club.
Malcolm McDonald on his No 7 500 cc Arial

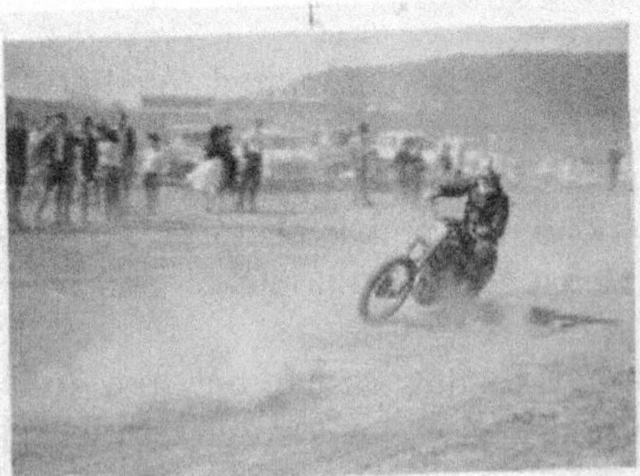

M.McDonald, 'The Flying Scotsman,' on his number 7

Other sports can have serious incidents when the unexpected takes a hand -

Aquatic Sports Injury.

I was on weekend Duty which came up every few months for the Honorary.
I had assisted the permanent Officers to carry out the set weekly routine tasks. Emptying and cleaning all cupboards, then checking and restocking if needed.

The phone bell rang, the senior answered the call then informed my permanent partner on the shift that the Cairns Harbour Board Pilot vessel would dock at number two wharf in about 20 minutes with a patient who had been injured with fish spear – the spear was still embedded in his leg.

This situation was quickly discussed and it was decided to take the new Ford Ranch wagon ambulance unit as this had the most room in the stretcher area.
We drove down to the wharf and parked close to the mooring capstan.
The trim Pilot boat was sighted in the Inlet and soon docked.
We boarded the vessel, examined our patient and obtained the history of the case.

The young man had been spear fishing with friends at Swain's reef for large reef fish such as Red Emperor, Cod or Sweetlip. He had swum for a time on the surface using a snorkel, saw a good sized Red, dived after it but missed the fish with his spear.

He then surfaced, loaded the speargun but decided to rest before the next foray, so he swam over to the dinghy, grasped the side with one hand and swung his speargun up and onto the rear seat. He then started to climb over the side into the boat.

Unfortunately the speargun fell off the seat due to the rocking of the boat as he swung his leg over the side, it discharged shooting the spear which entered his thigh immediately above his knee, travelled through his thigh muscle and stopped with the spearhead lying against the neck of the femur.
As he was fishing for large reef fish the spear was of 3/8 stainless steel with a 1/2 inch spearhead which had a retractable barb each side. The rounded swelling from the spearhead was quite obvious on/in the patient's hip with the spear shaft protruding a further 3 feet from his knee.

When in a semi-reclined position with the thigh supported and without movement, he had very little pain at this time.

All we could do at this point was to prepare the stretcher, and after instructing four helpers on how to support and lift the patient, we lifted him onto the stretcher then into the unit taking the utmost care to ensure the protruding spear shaft did not get bumped or caught on anything.
The patient was transported to the Cairns Base Hospital and straight to theatre.

Whatever sport or activity people enjoy, there are always precautions to be taken or rules to be obeyed so as to prevent injury or to reduce the risk. Do take due care.

THE RIGHT NIGHT.

When I started my honorary service at the Cairns centre there were 21 Honorary staff on roster, each on a specific night for duty, this allowed Honorary officers to work 2 duty nights out of 3 and provided 2 Honorary officers each night from 6pm to 10 pm.

My rostered night was a Tuesday, but I requested a Friday or Saturday night as soon as one became vacant, the reason being that more emergencies occurred on these nights.

When I was allotted a Saturday night I also requested permission to sleep at the centre to be available for duty until 8am Sunday as these were the busy nights.

This Saturday night in the late fifties had been fairly quiet from 6pm. with a couple of routine transports.

The main bit of excitement occurred when officers Wheat and his shift partner Andy filled one electric frypan with sausages and another with sliced onions, cooked the lot and then ate it all for supper. You see ambulance work can be stressful and officers had different ways of combating this problem.

A call came in about 1am from Edmonton that a lady was ill and required to see her Doctor. This person was a 'regular' in that she was an alcoholic and called on the ambulance frequently, a typical tragic case of a very gifted pianist who had succumbed to this unfortunate disease.

Col Wheat, the senior officer directed me to transport this case.

I placed an objection in that I did this extra duty to gain experience in emergency work not to do simple transports, and if anything serious occurred while I was away I requested that I be redirected, Col assured that this would be so.

Sure enough, as I was approaching the Doctors surgery with my self-induced ill patient, a message came over the radio. "car 14 arrived at scene", it was Andy Houser attending a road accident.

I was somewhat disconcerted and on disembarking my patient at the surgery, I called "free," but instead of being directed to support the other officer, I was directed to return to centre.

My adrenaline was flowing, so when I screeched to a stop at centre and reported, my feelings were apparent.

Officer Wheat who had given me much of his experience through training for ambulance competitions, knew my level of knowledge and skills, (and my enthusiasm), meet me with a calming hand and the information -

"A car has smashed into an electric light pole at Suicide Bend, the two occupants are injured and trapped."

" I want you to go out and assess the situation - you will find my mate walking around directing everybody, take no notice but go about the business of treating the injured, extricating them and transporting to Hospital - any problems have Andy radio me."

On arrival I found the car hard into the base of the pole, in fact the pole was splintered at the point of impact, with the top section leaning slightly and supported by the power lines attached.

The passenger's front door was wedged against a heavy hardwood railway fence post. The injured driver had been treated and removed to the first Ambulance unit, the injured passenger was still in the front passenger's seat, and appeared unconscious.
The Officer was directing helpers to chop away the hardwood post to gain access to the front passenger's door.

I made these observations on my approach, and I signalled to Andy that I had arrived and would check the patient in the smashed vehicle. I suggested that the C.R.E.B. be notified to make the power lines and pole safe, then dismissed that and gained access to the interior through the open rear door on the driver's side.

I leant over the injured patient, found him to be breathing, unconscious, pale, with a laceration to the left cheek over a probable fracture to the lower jaw, the examination of the lower limbs was awkward in the confined space but he also appeared to have a compound fracture to the right ankle, as I could feel a 'wetness' and swelling.

The dashboard was distorted inwards, the tail-shaft arch and floor were pushed up, and this prevented extrication over the driver's seat and out through the driver's door.

I then examined the seat and found it to be of the fully reclining type, [known then as a camping body], I got out, removed the stretcher from my unit, arranged this with a blanket and carry sheet, called for, and instructed a couple of bystanders on what I required.

I then re-entered the car, supported the patient, unscrewed the seatback holder and reclined the seat back fully.

By example I directed the helpers to support and lift the patient, and removed him out through the open driver's side rear door.

When this second patient was extricated, the other Officer left with the injured driver.

All officers were well aware of the limited staff so always cleared the scene as soon as possible if they were not required, so as to be available for the next emergency.

I re-examined my patient and treated him, immobilising his fractures and bandaging his wounds. He was then transported to the Cairns Base Hospital.

At the hospital the two casualties were identified as two of the hospital's Medical Interns who had been relaxing on their day off at the Yorkeys Knob hotel.

Dr Lester was the Medical Superintendent at that time and during his examination of one of the patients and receiving my report on the patient and the incident, asked further questions and become aware that I was an honorary officer.

He then demonstrated,[on his unconscious Intern], the method of jaw support to control airway obstruction from the tongue in the unconscious patient, and further, how the patients airway was immediately cleared and the patient breathed spontaneously when the jaw was supported and lifted.

That demonstration has never been forgotten, but such instruction by committed Medical officers was always given freely to Ambulance officers who showed an interest in their patients and in patient care.

Dr Lester was assisted by a Medical officer from the R.A.N., Dr. Cilento, who was updating on certain Medical procedures; later he and I had a smoke on the Hospital veranda and watched the sun come up over Trinity Bay.

This case demonstrated the need to assess the situation realistically as a practical exercise, identify the problem, examine with practised deliberation any proposed solution; decide on the action to be taken, and to prepare fully before acting.

Too often emotion is involved, ***and emotion is never a sound base for any practical decision,*** plus the desire to urgently free the trapped victim.

This may cause rescuers to sometimes see greater complications and difficulties than actually exist, but education and training allow clear objective assessment and action.

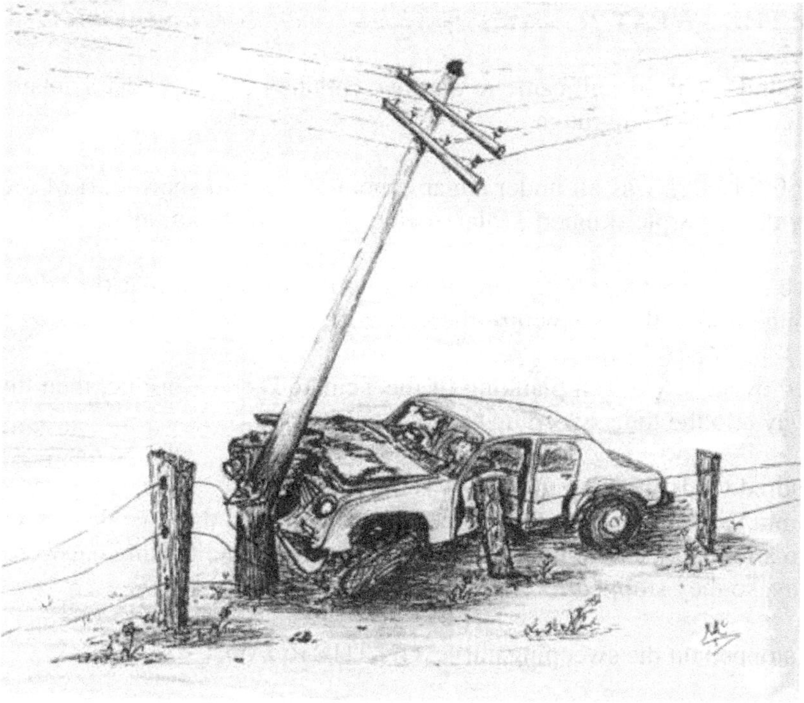

Drawing of the Suicide Bend accident.

All that being true, it can still make you 'sweat' as the next case will show.

WHY THE SWEAT ?

About mid-night the call came in that two cars had collided past Tomatoes creek on the back road to Kamarunga.

In 1960 this area was all under sugar cane, not the thin short stuff of today, but the stately thick, purple skinned Trojan variety that grew 9 foot tall.

Off we drove, roof lights flicking, (no rotating beacons at that time), siren wailing, weaving through the late picture-theatre traffic, (no TV either.)

Rattled over the wooden planking of the Tomatoes creek bridge, then turned off the highway into the long sweeping curve to the left.

A hundred yards further and there was the accident.
A Kombi van had ran into the rear of a car. We found that two groups were on their way to a mutual friend's home, but the occupants of the leading car were not sure of the way, so they stopped for the others to catch up.

They stopped on the sweeping curve, ON THE ROAD.

The high cane hid the car from the vehicle following, which on approaching at approx 60 mph, could not stop nor swerve in time and smashed into the rear of the first car.

The Kombi van had the engine mounted centrally and under the floor which left only the body metal in front of the driver and the bumper bar for protection.
This was virtually no protection at all, with the result that the front of the Kombi and the steering column were forced back into the cabin area.

The six other occupants of the two vehicles were mainly unhurt save for bruising and abrasions, but the driver of the Kombi was injured and trapped.

On climbing into the van I found the driver to be conscious and coherent, lying across the length of the front seat, with his right foot trapped by the bent steering column forcing his foot against the wall of the front seat support.

His right shoe was twisted up at the front and held to the floor.
The ankle as lacerated from the fractured bones of the lower ends of the tibia and fibula, bleeding was under primary natural control, the leg was bent at about 45 degrees to the ankle which was held upright by the column, the fractured ends of the bones were protruding.
The injury looked severe enough and had been open to infection from the time of being fractured - my first assessment was my patient might lose his foot.

I had to balance in the cabin, with my left foot on the seat and my right foot on the small running board, and had to twist down to reach the injury.
At first I simply splashed dilute antiseptic all over the injury then covered it with a clean dressing.

The permanent officer directed the extrication of the patient's foot using chains outside to pull the crushed front of the cabin forward, and a long crowbar through the door opening to lever the steering column forward.

During this procedure I remained in this strained, awkward position.

From the onset I had reassured my patient that we were there to assist him that everything was being done to extricate his foot; that he had injured his foot rather severely and that we would attend to his injuries and transport him to a Doctor and hospital as soon as we were able.

During the whole incident the patient was coherent, quiet, [unless asking or answering a question], and did not demonstrate being in pain.

In these situations one should expect anything, but as I worked on in this strained position, concentrating to protect the severe injury from further damage from the crowbar etc., my mind working on how I must support the unstable leg when the foot was freed, and also watching my patient for any deterioration.

He looked up at me in the reflected torch light and asked, **"WHAT ARE YOU SWEATING FOR MATE?"**
I was almost nonplussed but quickly replied, "I'm a bit out of condition."

The foot was freed, I carefully but firmly supported the injured ankle, the leg was raised onto the seat, laid on a dressing on a heavily padded wooden splint, further dressings over the injury, then the whole bandaged to the splint; further padding and a splint to the inside of the leg, broad bandages to thigh, knee and calf with a figure of 8 bandage to the foot.

Our patient was carried to the stretcher and transported to Cairns base hospital.

I can report that he did not lose his foot due to the severe damage sustained nor to infection, but was discharged some months later whole and hearty.

JULIA CREEK EXPERIENCES – 1962. Much to learn.

1962 - My philosophy was that all patients deserved the best in Emergency Pre-hospital Patient care available.
That is, Ambulance officers as the first equipped responder would administer 'up to date' treatments and procedures which would benefit the patient to:-

- restore vital functions,
- prevent any further deterioration,
- protect from further injury,
- thus reduce in- hospital and convalescence time.

This prompted me to be ever conscious of any improvement available for the administration of pre-hospital care and to be ever ready to listen and learn from anyone with respected knowledge in this field.

The Hospital Medico who received your trauma patients and the General Practitioner to whom you took the medical emergencies were always willing to tutor and pass on their knowledge to an officer who presented their patients with responsible treatments, gave a concise yet detailed verbal report on the situation and the patient's condition and showed a sincere interest in learning.

But, I had much to learn:

On being appointed as a permanent Ambulance officer to Julia Creek centre in March 1962, even though my training had provided me with the knowledge and skills to administer First-aid, I soon learned that 'the best of my ability' did not necessarily provide the optimum results from Pre-hospital Emergency Care even though I had high pass levels in First-aid, Home Nursing and Home Hygiene as well as good skills.

Later in the year the Superintendent directed me to an elderly patient who had had a 'fall' and was in pain.
On arrival the neighbour led me to the patient lying on the kitchen floor, pain to the left thigh and unable to stand.
On primary assessment I diagnosed a fractured femur.

I reassured my patient, explained that I was going to apply a special splint to his leg to control haemorrhage and pain so that I could transport him to hospital.

I collected the trilene for pain relief from the unit and the Thomas splint used to immobilise fractures of the femur.
This was an especial Thomas splint - a great nickel plated device with a padded ½ thigh ring, side bars, slides for leg length and a back plate. It had an adjustable footplate with an extension screw.
It was used for immobilisation of all fractures of the femur.

I adjusted the length of the splint beside the patient's leg - hip to footplate, then applied padding to the back-plate. Placed 4 x 3inch bandages beside the injured leg. I advised my patient on the use of the Trilene inhaler – to hold it firmly to his face and to inhale deeply to gain the best pain relief.

Once he had taken ten deep breaths I grasped his ankle with my left hand, took extension and with my right hand slid the splint under this leg so the padded half ring was firmly against his pelvis.

"Keep inhaling deeply now," I instructed.

I then strapped his foot to the footplate and adjusted the extension.
Folded triangular bandage around the top of the side bar and over the thigh to the other side to complete the 'ring' of the splint.
A quiet sigh of relief that all had gone to plan and training.

Figure of eight bandages along the leg and over the frame and I was ready to use the neighbour to assist to load my patient onto the stretcher, into the Ambulance and transported to the hospital.

On return to centre I proudly reported to Supt. Macklin my use of the Thomas splint and how well 'it' all went.
I was totally deflated by Ken's laconic reply. "Yeh! he'll probably be gone in three weeks!"
Ken explained: Even though the elderly patients benefited in the first instance from control of haemorrhage, immediate alignment of 'limb' and stability during transport, they still succumbed from complications of pneumonia or thrombosis due total bed rest and the level of Medical procedures available at the time.

This did not deter me as the realignment of the fractured bone and major blood vessels was the optimum goal to prevent further injury and blood loss and relieve pain. I used the basic Thomas splint for all fractures of the femur in future Centres.

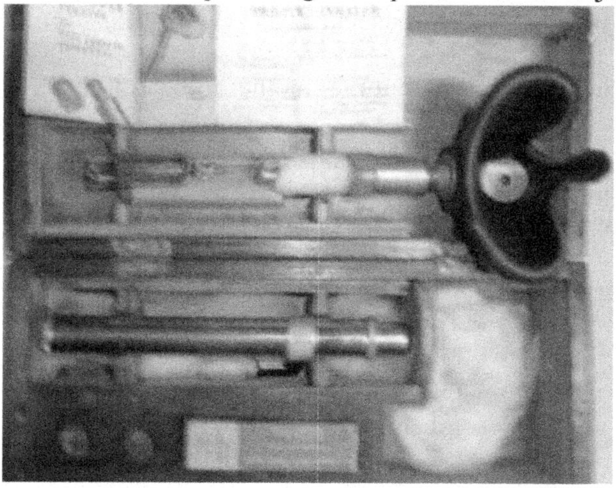

'The Trilene kit' demonstrating the components – phial, plunger and wool, facemask attached to cylinder top.

Complete cylinder in rack, trilene phial in packet, space with padding for facemask.

THE 'FIRST' MALCOLM.

The first time I delivered a baby was at Julia Creek, *and that was an occasion*. I had basic training in emergency childbirth and had maintained my studies, but had never witnessed an actual birth.

The Superintendent was away for the day when the call came in :-
"Mrs. Crawford is having a baby - come quickly"- " where?"- "in Coyne Street."

At last my first childbirth, or was it a panic call? well we'll soon know, I was excited - I told my wife, where I was going, double checked that I had the necessary kit, and drove off - my mind was working in top gear, going over the procedure for childbirth, and the questions to be asked.

That's the house - stop - out of the unit, kit in hand - up the front stairs - lady at the doorway - before I could speak, a hand pointed "in there" - I hurried in - the call said "having a baby." What would I find?

I found the expectant mother reclined on the bed seemingly in good spirits, totally relaxed and alone?? - this is not what I understood 'having a baby' depicted.

I stopped short, "how are you?" I asked, - - "good thanks," she replied.

That's not the right answer I thought, try again – "how are the pains?"

"Alright," she replied.

WRONG again for HAVING A BABY, try again - "how far are the pains apart?"

" Oooah, ju - ju - just a - mi-mi-min-ute," she gasped.

NOW that's the right answer - "I think we'd better check."

On checking I found the baby's head presenting, but the 'mother to be' still had her briefs on, causing a problem.

"LADY," I called, as I tried to control the birth of the neonate and endeavoured to get scissors out of my kit to cut away the briefs.

I cut the briefs between my fingers, while I instructed the other lady to get a couple of clean towels and to ring the Doctor.

The towels arrived as the babe was born - well, really I just caught him, because it was a premie birth, under weight and the second child.

The ‘cord’ was expelled following the babe, and what a cord it was!
It seemed to be so thick, and just kept coming and coming!

Of course it was simply a fully engorged cord, seem by me, for the first time.

The baby cried - I smiled - the mother spoke - “what is it?” - “a boy” - Doctor Duggan arrived.

He then took over and clamped, then cut the cord, and a pad and bandage was lightly applied, the babe checked, then wrapped in a ‘bunny rug.’

I thought this was the greatest thing since electric light - everyone congratulated everyone on a job well done.

The delivery of a new babe into the world is one of the most rewarding experiences for anyone, a moment to be treasured.

Of course the child was christened ‘Malcolm.’

STATION VISITS.

After I had been in the town for a while, Superintendent Ken Macklin tasked me with collecting subscriptions from the station properties in our district.

This entailed travelling through a section of the district, calling at each station on the way, stopping overnight at an appropriate station, continuing on each day until that section was completed.

This not only ensured financial support but it also kept ambulance contact with the people in this vast and sparsely populated region. By travelling through the area I would learn the roads, tracks and property situations.

This was a another new experience for me and an important instructional one at that, for this way of life was an unknown factor to me and if I was to serve these people I had to learn quickly, so as to understand and communicate with them with ease and assurance.
On calling at one station in the 4WD Land Rover Ambulance, I soon found these people had a typical sense of humour.

I had talked with the Grazier for some time, given him the local news, [the latest and most topical was the new young Ambulance officer who had recently arrived], I had diplomatically introduced the subject of why I had called, this had been consciously ignored by the grazier.

He carried on with local issues, sizing me up all the while, which didn't take much to rate me as pretty raw to the west.

At last he said,(looking at me sideways) "so you're after donations for the ambulance eh!", pause - "well, I always give a bale of wool!"

In my innocence, I courteously replied "thank you, we appreciate your generous assistance."
With that, he came straight back at me with," **but you must take it now!"**

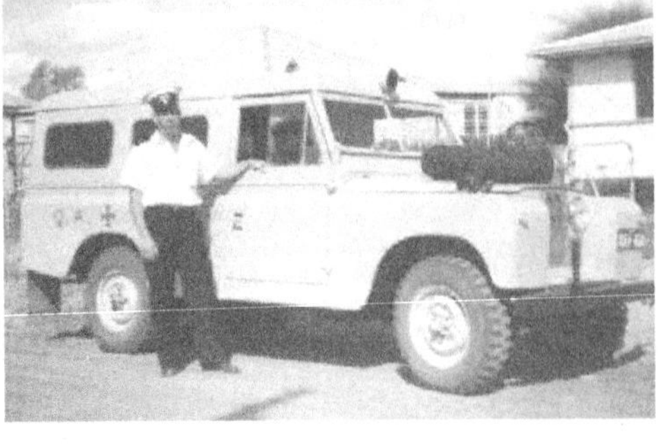

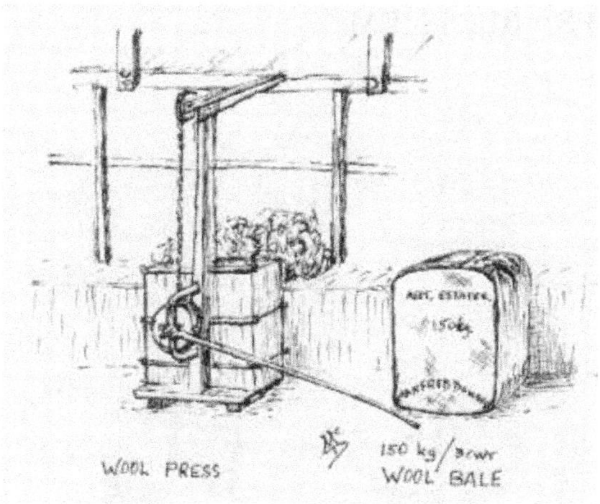

Sketch of Manual Wool Press

'Brother, what was this, guns at ten paces?' it was obvious he was taking me on.
I wasn't green enough not to realise this or to know how big a bale of wool was,(and these were the old bales not the reduced size of today).

"Right" I said, trying to sound matter-of-fact and walked over to the unit.
I put whatever equipment I could on the front passenger seat and floor, unhooked the stretcher and tied it to the side of the rear compartment, then backed up to the wool shed, heaved, pushed, and shoved the closest bale into the back of the unit, it just fitted neatly.

I again thanked the grazier for his generosity, gave him a smile and drove off.

To this day I don't know if he thought the bale would fit or not, but there was no way I would have left without it.
This was typical western humour and meeting it was the expected thing, whether you bettered it or not was not important, the important thing was *'to give it a go'*.

I found a welcome hospitality wherever I called, for these people appreciated the Ambulance service, but they also accepted each person on their merits as they found them.

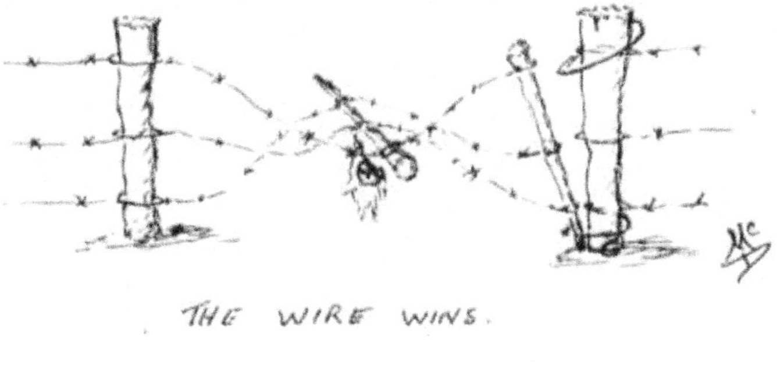

STATION GATES – BLESS 'EM.

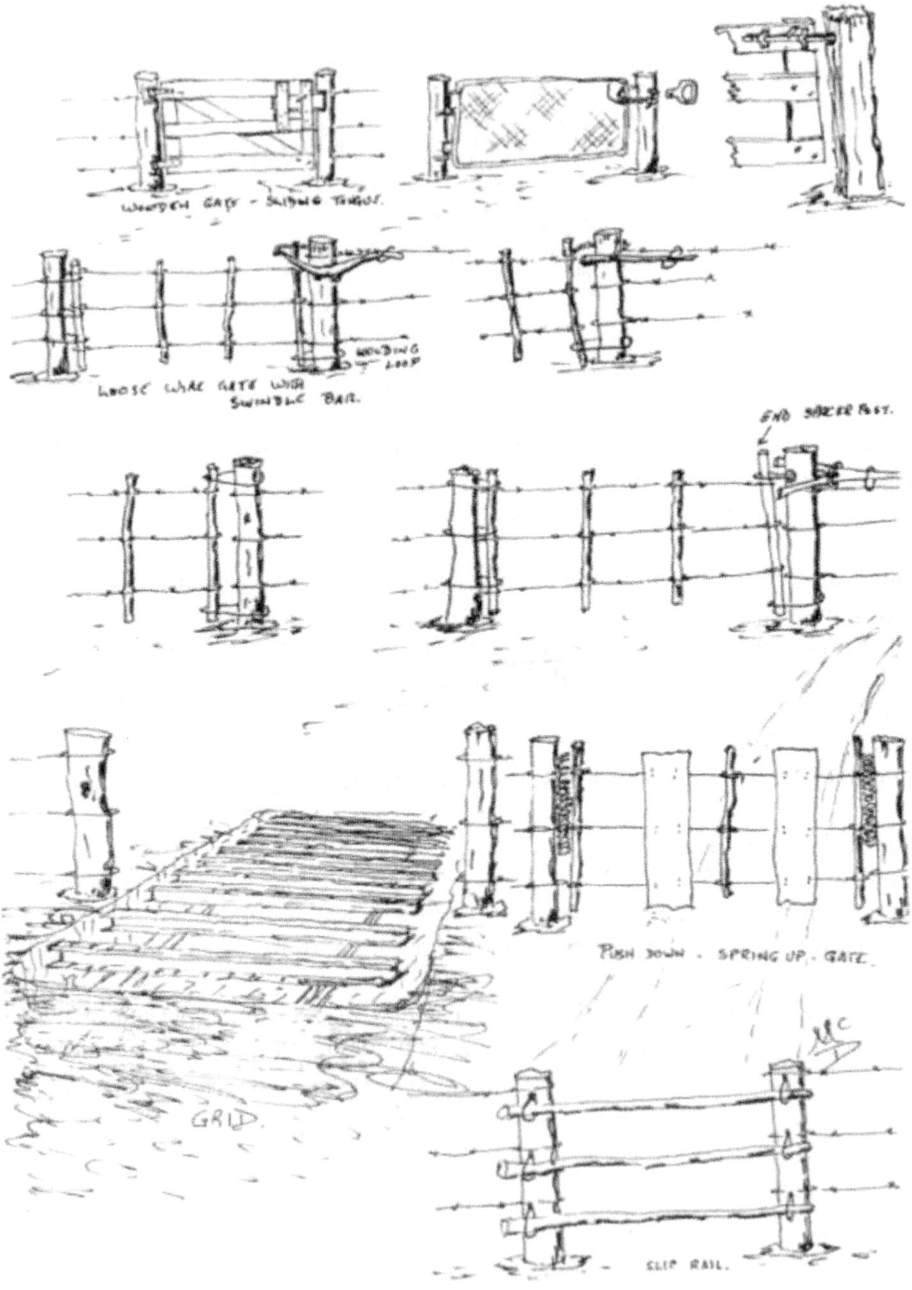

Station Gates.

ONLY THE BEST WILL DO.

I was called to an outstation of Toolebuk station, southwest of McKinley to attend to David Hogarth the overseer, who had been thrown and injured.
The trip to the outstation was about 100 miles and on reaching my patient, I found him conscious, slightly pale, resting in the shade, supporting his left arm.

The history of the case was that my patient had been riding the far paddock looking for strays, when a large sand goanna had reared up at the horse and hissed, spooking it and causing David to fall sideways onto his outstretched hand.

I prepared bandage rings for each shoulder, padding for each axilla and the extension bandage to pull on the two rings so as to apply extension to the left shoulder to realign the collar bone and immobilise the fracture.

I reassessed the injury, [the end of the overriding broken bone was obvious under the skin, there was 100 miles to travel to hospital], and decided I required a special pad to take the pressure but to relieve discomfort, but what ?

Yes, I know just the thing, I rummaged through a cupboard, found what I required, an ideal round firm pad with some resilience.

I lay the centre of a narrow bandage over this firm pad lying between the shoulder blades.
I then took each end and threaded them through the respective left and right bandage ring at each shoulder. These ends were returned over the central pad and tied in a half knot.

With an end of this extension bandage in each hand I applied steady outward pressure which was transferred over the fulcrum of the centre pad as a pulley action on the shoulder rings thus steadily pulling the shoulder joint back and pulling the clavicle outward until it was in line and not overriding.
The half knot was twisted to hold from slipping and a further knot was applied to hold this knot firm.

I applied a sling to the left arm to support and immobilise it, then examined my work.

Yes, the padding was firm but soft, large, but moulded to the body, the ideal padding for those rough trips - THE DUNNY ROLL DOES THE JOB.
Yes the new roll of toilet paper was just the thing as a pad for the extension required for a fractured collar bone.

We both had a cup of tea, then set off for the long trip to Julia creek.

THE OTHER SIDE TO SAVING LIVES.

The Doctors role was very rewarding and interesting, and he was usually seen in 'whites' at the surgery or at the hospital, and would be with other responsible citizens and graziers at golf or to the front at local functions, but, *there was another side*, a Doctor sometimes has cause to attend to the deceased as well, and he does this in a professional manner.

I received a call from Doc Duggan one Sunday morning, "Malcolm, wonder if you could help me, the wards man is away this weekend and I have to do a post mortem, would you assist me?"

Well, what do you say to that, "yes Doctor, when and where," I replied.

The thing was that in Queensland, the Hospitals Act was so written that no ambulance was to carry a 'dead' body, that is a person who had been certified as dead by a qualified Medical officer. This was a sensible clause in that Ambulances were not 'put out of use' in this manner, and were thus always available to administer to the sick and injured.

So this was another first for me, I had not even witnessed a post mortem before, so it was to be a sharp learning curve.

When I arrived at the Hospital Doc Duggan took me to the morgue where the body of a man, about 40 years of age, was lying on the dissecting table covered with a sheet.

This had the appearance of misadventure, in that the Police had been notified that a person who had been reported missing yesterday, had been found in the flooded creek last night, but, as this was a case of sudden death, then a post mortem had to be carried out to identify the actual cause of death, so here we were.

A post mortem is carried out in similar manner to any surgical operation, but in this case the organs of the body are exposed and examined for any abnormality or damage, the main ones being the brain, heart, lungs and stomach.

I was assisted in handling this foreign situation by the professional manner of Doctor Duggan, he carried out his examination as a teaching exercise, where, as he exposed certain organs he described their structure and role, as well as what he had to look for.

It was a most educational experience and invaluable in the knowledge I gained, which would assist me in understanding injuries and the effects of illness.

I assisted the Doctor in passing instruments and in using the special oscillating electric saw to remove the top of the cranium to allow him to examine the brain for injury.

The problem for me was that there is a certain smell about a morgue which insinuates itself into the olfactory nerves and the subconscious.

On returning home I changed in the laundry and then soaped and showered myself a few times, but I could still smell the morgue.

For months after, and even an odd time in years to be, I would still recall that smell when I inhaled other odours, one being roasting pork, so for a time I did not eat certain foods.

THE LONGEST NIGHT.

This was the Centenary of the Cobb and Co. Coach Company, and to celebrate the occasion the Cobb and Co. coach was running again, from Cairns to Melbourne, along the inland route.

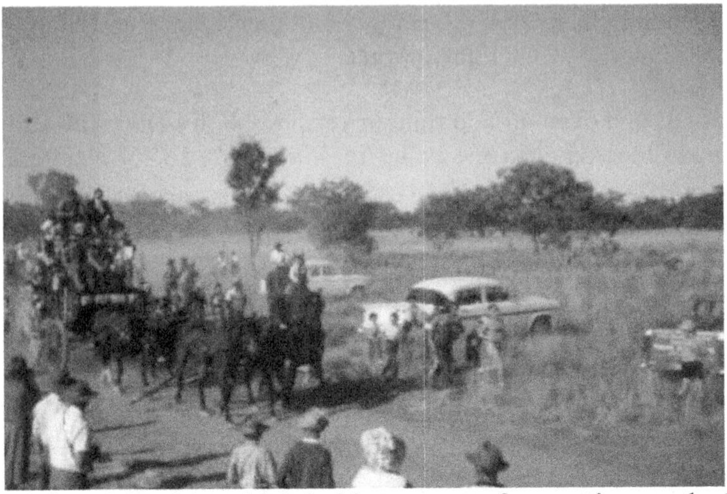

What a spectacle, of the driver high in his seat, one foot resting on the brake lever with six - in – hand. Six magnificent horses at full gallop, something to remember.

The coach was to arrive about mid-day and water that night at Combo Water hole below Kynuna, the famous water hole of Banjo Patterson's Waltzing Matilda.
There would be entertainment and a Bush Dance that night.

Everybody who was anybody, would be there, not the Bearer though, he had to mind the fort.

As it was only 75 miles away, I suggested Val might drive down with the children and a friend Pat Case the wife of the Shire Council Overseer.
In the Inland you had to make your own entertainment, so 75 miles (120 km.) to travel for an event was nothing.

People travelled for hundreds of miles to attend, the Bush Airstrip was surrounded by all type of light aircraft, the Flying Surgeon and the Flying Doctor were there as was the Doctor from Julia creek, the Ambulance Superintendent, Shire clerk etc., etc.

The day was quiet, everyone had left town.
The peace was broken when the radio crackled to life at 6 pm.
It was the Super calling for a Report.
I could only say, “all is quiet.”

Dr. Duggan came on the air next and requested a phone hook-up with the Hospital, and relayed instructions through me for certain treatments for patients, then the Flying Doctor asked if there were any messages for him.

The Superintendent concluded with the info that all were signing off and would be attending the night festivities.

I only had time to check that all was in place before I went for dinner when the phone rang. It was 20 minutes past 6pm. It was the Overseer of the station below Claravale, about 300 km's NNE of Julia creek.

His 12 year old daughter had just been kicked in the head by a horse, it was too late for any light aircraft to fly her out, so they would start for Julia creek as soon as they could and asked if I would come and meet them.

I took full particulars - unconscious, large scalp wound at the back of the head, they would travel down the only track from the station till it met the track from Esmeralda, and expected to meet me after that.

I rang the Police Sergeant for directions and detail about the track.

Sergeant said, "from Bunda Bunda you've got Mullungera turn off to your left a mile up, and Savannah Downs again off to your left another 12 mile to the North, straight after that is Saxby Downs turnoff to the right, and 25 miles on to the junction of Claravale and Esmeralda tracks, Claravale is the left fork."

"What's the track like?" I asked.
" It's different above Bunda, you'll have sandy soil through the dry flood channels from the tributaries of the Norman, and could be a bit damp if you get as far as the Norman itself.
The track runs through scrub country after the first ten mile or so, just follow the heavy wheel track."

"Thanks Sarg," piece of cake I thought, HA!

I checked the 4WD long wheelbase Land Rover, Val had arrived home by this, so I called her for sandwiches and a thermos, made sure the spare jerry can was full of petrol and secure, drove the unit from under the centre and attached the long range aerial extension to the spring mounted normal aerial, thus adding another six foot to it.

I drove out of the Centre at about 7 pm that Saturday night.

I made good time over the 'main dirt road' from The Creek to Nelia and on to Bunda Bunda, but soon after leaving Bunda the road surface and the terrain changed.

The surface was sandy, the road wound its way along any available high ground beside the creek beds, I used the 4WD when I crossed dry sandy channels - reflection of eyes of a fox or dingo - further along the track twisted its way through stunted scrub country.

The night was pitch black, and driving through the stunted scrub was like driving through a torturous twisting tunnel that never ended.

Stop, open one of those jolly gates, drive through, get out and close the damn thing, then on again.
I lost track of time as I continued driving, the going was slow because of the sandy track and the twisting road, it was simply follow the two deep wheel ruts as quick as you could,[there's an injured child somewhere ahead], wrench of the wheel to miss a tree when the track took a sharp turn.

Munch on a sandwich to stay alert and to keep up the energy, stop, get out to relieve yourself, be brave and take two steps away from the unit (not too far, because by this I wasn't sure where the hell I was, I was now at the point of **HOPING** that I was still on the right track).

Good, this must be the fork to Claravale and Esmeralda, (I hope) took the track to the left. Some miles further on I am suddenly confronted with car lights, **THANK GOODNESS**.

The stunted scrub and twisting track had concealed any light until we actually met on the single vehicle track.

First check the patient, conscious but dozing, [easily rouseable], there was a rough towel bandage to the head, [soaked with blood], bleeding controlled by the bandage and natural clotting.
I transferred the patient onto a stretcher and into the Ambulance, where I assessed my patient more fully, then removed the towel and placed sterile gauze swabs and ample padding over the area and firmly bandaged over it.

We then had a quick 'cuppa' to lift our energy levels and turned for the return journey to Julia Creek and the Hospital.

A couple of stops to reassess my patient, resting quietly, [all's well] - ate the last sandwich, carry on.
First light is a magic time driving through the inland, all is quiet, a cool gentle breeze, the light is soft as it strengthens, grazing kangaroos lift their heads in curiosity at your approach.
A plains turkey lazily lifts out of the Flinders grass on effortless slow wings.

Bunda Bunba station was a welcome sight at about 6am after sunrise, then on past and heading for 'The Creek.'

I arrived at the Hospital at 8 am on the Sunday morning, the trip had taken 13 hours from leaving the Centre at 7pm., the night before.

Back to the centre to refuel the unit, wash it, and dust it out inside, restock it and put it away before going home next door, checking if any cases were in transit or just came in, then - HORIZONTALISE - what luxury.

Another day AND LONG NIGHT ends.

RECREATION AND SPORT – we assist in many ways!

The feral pig numbers were excessive and they destroyed native and cultivated pasture extensively.
They were not just scavengers but also devoured new lambs and whatever was within their range so Graziers were pleased if responsible people came onto the property to deplete numbers.
One could not be complacent as a mature wild pig was a very dangerous animal and would charge on sight or smell of a human interloper.

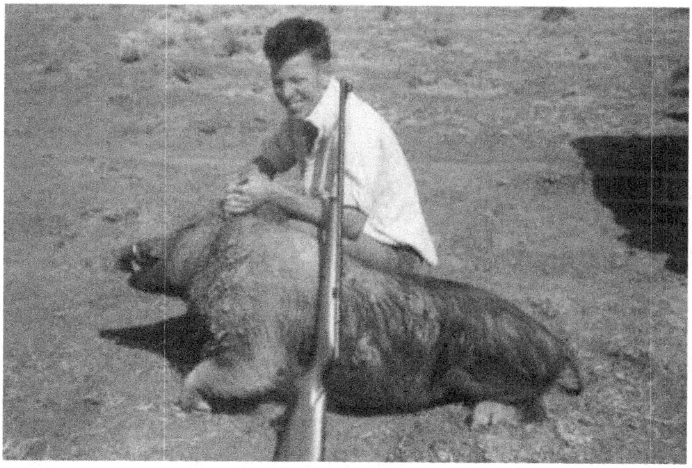

1963 - we assist with the feral problem.

QATB ROCKHAMPTON IN 1964.

On my appointed to QATB Rockhampton in 1964 I gained much experience but came to the opinion that the only way to progress was to gain a position where I would be able to decide on the level of service provided.
Although Rockhampton was a good Centre there was a lack of leadership and direction so that we sometimes took things into our own hands:-
My shift partner Graham Buxton, myself and Everard Smith the mechanic made aspirators ('suckers') for the Rockhampton units from those I had seen at the QATB Brisbane Centre.

To this end I volunteered for duty as an Air Attendant on the Central Qld. Aerial Ambulance conducted by QATB Rockhampton.

NIL FEET -
On arriving for duty at 8am at Rocky centre, I was called to the office of the Deputy Superintendent Neville Fraser, who in his indubitable fashion, informed me, "son, you'll be flying an infant down to Brisbane today in the Aerial Ambulance, the Pilot has left for the airport, get your gear and report out there."

"Where from Neville? What's wrong with the patient?" I asked.
"It's a Boy Scout job son, you'll pick up a nurse and the patient outside Biloela," Neville was never long, or strong, on detail. Neville was ever the 'Boy Scout.'

Out to the airport, checked the aircraft equipment, oxygen cylinders and stretcher security, then reported to Ralph Phillipson the pilot at the Flight room where he was completing his flight plan before submitting same.

All's completed. Taxi out, final checks. Ralph received permission from the tower, rev of motor and down the strip, and lift off.
Then up into the blue sky and onto the bearing for the Biloela bush strip, a lovely day for a flight.

We landed on the bush strip outside Biloela, and Ralph taxied the Aerial Ambulance over to the waiting Ambulance car and cut the engine.

I walked over to the open Ambulance car and reported to Superintendent Fred Leader.
An infant was in a humidicrib in the back of the ambulance, a nurse in attendance. I asked the Superintendent what was the patient's condition and what was required?

I received the abrupt (English) accented reply to a junior officer, "just get the oxygen ready in the plane," and he turned away to take the humidicrib out of the ambulance.
I hurried over to the aircraft, entered and readied the stretcher straps to secure the

crib, attached a length of oxygen tubing to the supply line and turned on the main oxygen cylinder.

I warned the pilot that we would be carrying a patient on oxygen and that I would be opening the line when the patient was on board - precautions must be taken when oxygen is present in the aircraft.

The Super arrived at the door and handed the crib inside, as I leant over to take and lift the crib onto the stretcher I noticed that the infants face was heavily cyanosed, I stopped, grabbed the oxy tube and attached it to the crib and turned the oxygen on, no worry as to the rate, just ON.

I placed the crib onto the stretcher, secured it, called the nurse, then adjusted the oxygen rate to the correct setting.

I discussed the patient's condition with the Nurse who informed me that the patient had a heart deformity which required specialist surgery within the next few days, otherwise its future was doubtful.

Once the patient and Nurse were on board the Pilot started the engine and commenced his pre flight check, I made sure the nurse was comfortable, then instructed her on the fittings and equipment in the aircraft, even though the patients main requirement was the oxygen, the nurse having all other needs in her kit.

I moved to the front seat beside the Pilot, he asked about the condition of the patient to which I gave a full report.

On hearing of the patient's reaction when the crib had no oxygen for only a couple of minutes, and well aware that the aircraft was not pressurised, he asked, "what height then?"

I replied "that due to the problem of the patient's heart, anything that put extra demand on it was detrimental, such as reduced oxygen or alteration in atmospheric pressure."

" I'm going to declare this flight a Mercy Mission and request permission to fly at nil feet," the pilot informed me.
He then contacted Flight control at Rockhampton and informed them of the status of the flight and his flight plan.
They gave permission to fly at nil feet.

As Ralph prepared for takeoff he said, "we'll fly direct to the coast following the railway line, then follow the coast flying over the sea to the mouth of the Brisbane river, then up the river to the airport."
The route chosen gave no obstructions, was level all the way and was the most

direct. Ralph had a number of possible routes recorded that he could use if a situation such as this actually occurred.

We took off, **NIL FEET was BELOW FIVE HUNDRED FEET.**

The Nurse had been occupied with checking the gauges and settings of the humidicrib for temperature, humidity and oxygen rate, and she was taking and recording the infant's vital signs when I informed her of our flight plan, she nodded her approval and continued.

I was glued to my seat and thrilled to the core at what I was experiencing when the Nurse looked up from her tasks - I heard a gasp from her because we were flying **THROUGH A RAILWAY CUTTING.**

Both she and I now appreciated what nil feet really meant.

What a wonderful flight that was, the route made it safer than most conventional flights, the low height made it spectacular for us and totally balanced for the infant with no changes in atmospheric pressure at all.

As we flew over the sea and along the coast people fishing in small boats would look up at us, see the Aerial Ambulance markings and wave to us, I believe they understood that we were flying low because of a very ill patient and were wishing us well.

We landed at Brisbane airport without incident, an Ambulance with two officers was waiting for us. When we parked and the Pilot switched off the engine the ambulance was driven onto the apron close to the aircraft.

I immediately alighted, went to the Officers and reported on the patient's condition then instructed them to unclip an oxygen cylinder with regulator from their Ambulance, and to take it to the Humidicrib in the aircraft.

I re-entered the aircraft, informed the Nurse of my arrangements, them uncoupled the aircraft oxy line, attached the line from the oxygen cylinder from the ambulance and turned it on at the correct setting then assisted in transferring the crib with its precious patient from the aircraft to the ambulance unit. The patient's condition did not alter in the slightest.

The Nurse went in to the hospital with the patient so as to give a handover report, Ralph and I checked and restocked our respective areas of responsibility, then had lunch.

All was ready for takeoff when the Ambulance returned with the Nurse, so off we went on our return flight but flying the conventional route at the normal light aircraft height of about 7000 feet.

The infant was operated on a couple of days later, the op was successful and the babe returned to its much relieved and thankful parents some time later.

Years later I learned that the patient was a Biloela Ambulance Officer's daughter – great stuff.

So ended another voluntary duty, yes, qualified air attendants had to volunteer to fly in the Aerial Ambulance, as there was no wage allowance for this nor was there an award provision.

Any officer willing to provide this important service to the people of the outback and to serious cases from the Rockhampton Base Hospital had to sign as volunteers. A large number of the staff would not fly until extra payment was awarded as an Aerial Attendant allowance in the 1970's.

BELOW: the Central Queensland Aerial Ambulance Cessna 128 from the retrieval and the later more modern craft with officers Buxton and McDonald.

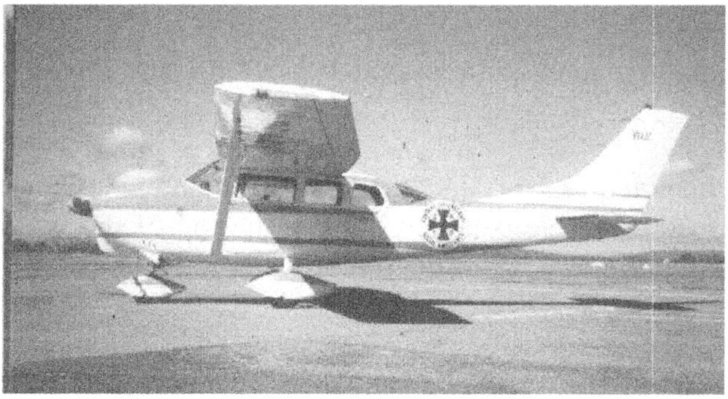

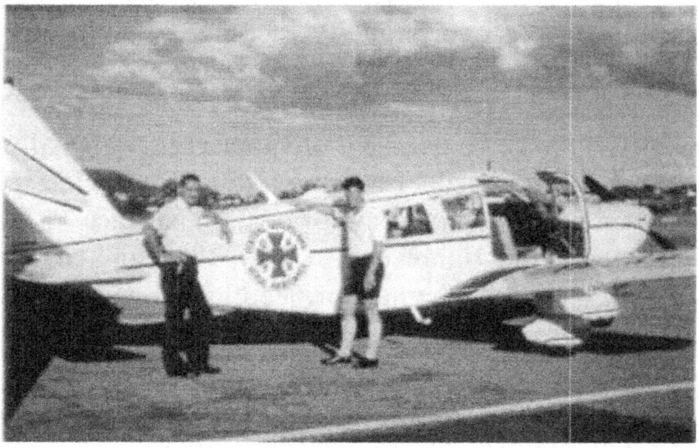

MY BROTHER'S name is MALCOLM:

It was a normal Saturday afternoon for Rocky Ambulance, reasonably quiet, some showers earlier, so Graham and I had been able to complete our domestic duties for that shift.

About four thirty pm. the phone rang in the Control room and was answered by the Senior Bearer, Allan Brown.

I was the running man on this four to midnight shift so I stepped out of the duty room to ascertain the type of call being received and to be available if it was an emergency.

Allan replaced the handset and called," Malcolm, a case to be done."

I reported to the Control room.
Allan said, "I've just had a call for an ambulance to take a sick women to hospital, but there's something fishy about it, I don't know what, but it doesn't ring true , I couldn't get any real information, anyway go round and check it out, I'll be by the radio if you need help."

He gave me the details of name, address, and I drove off and duly arrived at the residence.

It was a large, old, unpainted Queenslander, with a front and side veranda, railings and lattice panels. It had a double panelled door at the top of the wide stairs, one tread of which was missing, there was a puddle of water in front of the bottom step, a drizzle of rain in the air.

A matronly lady opened the front door and beckoned that this was the house.

I alighted, reached for my kit and hurried through the drizzle, jumped the puddle, hopped over the missing step, stepped onto the veranda.

I looked at this motherly figure for information:-
She closed the door - a three and a two year old appeared at the hallway door -
" inside you pair," they disappeared - I heard a movement behind me - turned to see a women lying on a bed with an expression of pain on her face - I looked back at the lady - she nodded toward the figure on the bed, then looked at the reappearing children - shooed them back into the hallway - followed and closed the house door after her.

I stepped to the bed, smiled down at the women," now what's the trouble?" I asked, a little voice replied, " I'm pregnant and the babies coming."

Well there you are I mused. Aloud I said "you'll be alright" and took her hand, "but I'll radio the centre for assistance, won't be a moment," I released her hand and walked to the door.

Once through the door I galvanised into action, I stepped down the stairs three at a time, jumped the puddle, wrenched open the car door, snatched the radio hand piece.

"Car 12A, I request assistance at this residence, confinement - send Graham Buxton!" I got the reply, "message received."

I waited for no more, picked up the obstetric kit, raced back up the stairs, sudden stop on the top step, quiet walk to the bed, quiet deep breaths to slow the fast heartbeats.

As I opened the kit and arranged its contents at the end of the bed I asked, "now, are you nine months, and how are the pains?"

"Yes, the baby's due, but no one knew about it, and I went to work this morning, the water broke before and I asked Mum to call you," this information came tumbling out with relief.

"Now how are the pains ?"

"It's started," she grimaced.

" O'k nothing to worry about, I've delivered babies before, so everything's going to be alright," I said as I reached for an absorbent underlay.
"Now I'm going to check you to assess the baby's progress, so just do what I say and help me to help you."

I didn't have to say much at all, the lady was fully aware and assisted me to place the underlay under her buttocks, but when I tucked her dress up I looked at - A PAIR OF STEPINS - damn!

Now I really went into top gear, for my patient had given an obvious look and movement of bearing down, " pant, pant for me," I instructed, and reached for my scissors from the open kit beside me.

A gust of wind, from the uncertain weather, **'BANG'** slammed the front door.

I cut the stepins away, tore off the briefs, THE BABY WAS BEING BORN, this was her third child.

The head was presenting - hair, occipital - good normal birth - "you're right, pant now, pant," the head was born with my palm controlling and supporting it.

Movement on the stairs - looked up as Graham reached the top step - door shut, yale lock, -

" **LADY** " I called.

" It's O'k, my mate has arrived to assist us," I told my patient as I checked for the cord, yes it's around the neck.

" **LADY OPEN THE DOOR PLEASE** ," I called out again as I hooked a finger under the cord to ease it over the neonates head - quick look up - had to smile at what I saw - I looked down again at the continuing birth process.

When I looked up I saw my mate locked outside looking through the lattice work.

" Now a nice bearing down," I encouraged as I saw the next contraction start - turn of the head as the first shoulder presents - finger in the axilla - gentle lift - second shoulder born -- “that's the way, you're doing fine,” - supporting the head and neck - final contraction - other hand under the babe as it is born - cord following.

" Well done" I said to the mother," it's a boy," as I supported the child in the correct ankle hold and checked the airway for foreign material - **" Wwaarr"** - what a wonderful sound, then 'yes well done ' I said to myself as my heart filled with happiness to be part of this wonderful event.

On cue, the new Grandmother opened the hallway door and stepped onto the veranda, I nodded towards the front door where Graham was still standing outside, she opened it and Graham hurried in.

With Graham assisting I double clamped the umbilical cord, cut the cord, then dressed the end and placed a binder over this and around the babe, wrapped babe in a clean towel and gave it to the Mother to suckle.

I noted the distance of the cord externally from the mother,[for later indication that the placenta had separated], and we then started to tidy up.
As we worked I quietly obtained the history of this case.

The new mother was a married lady with two children, but problems had arisen in the marriage and she and her husband had separated.

The lady had moved to her widowed mother’s home and obtained a job as a shop assistant.

She had still maintained some contact with her separated husband.

She had told no one of her condition, and had not consulted a Doctor at any time.

She had worked that morning, this explained the step-ins.

I asked to which hospital she would like us to transport her, but she was most definite that she wanted to stay at home, she did accept our proposal that we ask the Government Medical officer to call.

We tidied up, then carried the lady inside to a bedroom and left. We were of the opinion that she would probably change her mind as nature took its course.

As soon as we arrived back at the Centre I phoned the Government Medical officer and explained the situation fully, he was about to be seated for dinner, but true to his calling agreed to attend the new mother immediately.

Graham had been busy on the other phone, ringing his wife and a couple of friends for any spare nappies or baby clothes they might have to give to our previous patient.

A couple of hours later the Doctor rang and Allan put me on the phone. The Doctor had attended to the lady but requested that we call and inform her that he wanted her to be admitted to the Base hospital for a couple of days.

We discussed the situation with the Senior bearer who agreed for Graham to leave and collect the spare babies gear he had organised, and for me to meet him at our patients home.

We presented ourselves to the patient who was most pleased to see us, firstly because the after effects of the birth were setting in, and especially for the gift of nappies and baby clothes Graham had organised.

She was quite willing now to go to hospital, so we organised things, carried her by stretcher to the unit, and transported her and babe to hospital.

As we turned to leave the ward she called us back and asked if we would mind if she had the baby christened Malcolm Graham after us, MIND, we walked on air out of the hospital.

SEQUEL:

One would expect the story to end there but some months later the annual Ambulance Carnival was being conducted in the park opposite the centre.

Graham and I were selling tickets at a stall when a voice said," hello fellers, look what I've got." We both looked at the speaker and there was our previous patient nursing our namesake, beside her were two young boys.

Of course we stopped and went and talked and had a nurse, and in doing so I turned to the youngest boy an asked," is this your baby brother ?", very proudly he replied, "yes," with a twist of his body in shyness.

"What's his name?" I asked.

"Malcolm," came the reply as I well knew.

"Well I never" I said, "my name is Malcolm too."

He got most upset, he turned to his mother and exclaimed, "he can't have Malcolm's name, *that's his name not the man's*."

Oh well, instead of making friends I'd upset the lad, so we said our farewells and left it to Mum to explain things, what a story it would make, and of course it has.

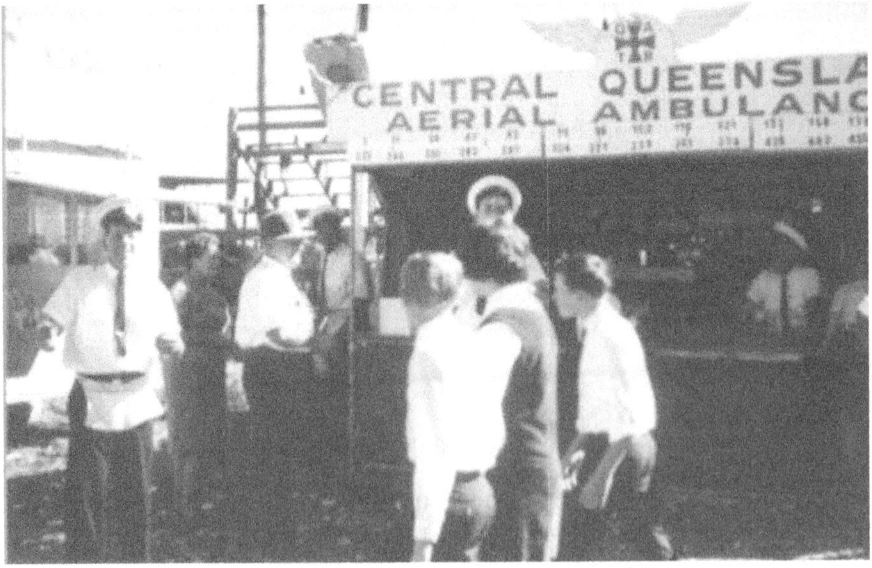

WOWAN QATB 1969:

In 1969 I was fortunate to serve at the one man station of Wowan where the resident Doctor and Medical Superintendent of the Mt. Morgan Hospital 25 miles away conducted fortnightly clinics.
The Ambulance carried certain medications and drugs under the Superintendent's responsibility and control through the Medical Superintendent of Mt. Morgan Hospital.

Self study: Wowan:
Dr. Wilson in Cairns had loaned me a copy of Pye's Surgical Handicraft, a medical textbook to read when I was recuperating from a bout of infectious Hepatitis I contacted in Julia Creek.
I now purchased a copy and other textbooks and applied myself to study.

Wowan conducted a 'Doctors Day' every 2 weeks when the Mt. Morgan Hospital Superintendent with the right to Private Practice attended.
The Centre held drugs for his use when he prescribed medication for a patient who attended at his clinic.
The only drugs and injections I had handled previously were for veterinarian treatment of our milking goats and pig on our Nerimbera farm.

The Centre Drug cupboard was a real challenge which I had to check and absorb quickly. The first chance I had to talk with Doctor John Mc Cosker in his Surgery I raised the subject of the Drug cupboard and how I needed something to assist me to quickly familiarise myself with its contents.
Doctor stood and reached over to his bookshelf and took down a large black covered volume, it was the previous year's Pharmacopoeia.

This tome was segregated into the various body systems, Respiratory, Vascular, Digestive etc, then sub headed for the ailment.
The recommended drug/drugs were listed with their properties, effects and contra indications. Every drug on the market was listed in its relevant reference for prescribing with the description of the tablet/capsule/solution with numbered colour plates for identification.

I studied each drug held by the Centre so that I was familiar with all.

This reference volume was invaluable for me in my dispensing drugs on behalf of the Doctor, for I would always double check on the prescription:-
(1) that I had followed orders.
(2) for any contra indications.
(3) that the patient did not have any condition that would cause a side effect.

This protected, the patient, the Doctor and myself.

In 1969 some drugs held: -
Topical applications i.e. decicain drops, Neosporin drops and ointment, cerumol drops. Ointments of ichthamol, ung-vita, butesin pictrate, Benadryl etc.
Tablets: penicillin PVK, ephedrine, sulphaquanidine, phenergan, nembudein etc.
Solutions: kaolin and OPI, etc.
Diagnostic test strips of flurostrip, clinistix, albustix etc.
I.M.I. of anti-tetanus and specific injections of procaine penicillin were 'as required.' Later: lasix, bronchepherin and phenergan.

The patient's permission for administering an injection was always requested, and always received.
By adhering to strict procedures I gained and maintained a trust with not only the Doctor, Chemist and patients but also with the Medical Specialists in Rockhampton.

Upgrade: In about 18 months time much of the tablets and capsules were replaced by I.M.I. therapy solutions as prescribed by the next Medical Superintendent of Mt. Morgan Hospital [with the right of private Practice], Dr. Gary Martin.
Attendance at Stage I QASB Training school gave instruction and experience of injections and cannulation.

Dr. Martin 'sized me up' after a week or so, then upgraded the drugs with a few injections for specific emergencies, for, as he said, "if you attended a genuine asthma attack or allergic reaction in the district, the patient would probably be dead before you reached me at Mt. Morgan."

I then carried IMI injections of lasix, bronchepherin and phenergan with me for emergent calls.

At the Centre I also had stocks of anti tetanus, and various anti-biotic injections. Other medications, e.g. :- abbocillin, neotracin, streptomagma, tetrex, pensig, teledrin, ancolan and various others, all in the locked cupboard and recorded in the drug book.

This gave an out-patient facility and immediate availability of specialised emergency care to the residents of the Wowan district under the supervision and authority of the Medical Superintendent of Mt. Morgan Hospital - a system that was practical and cost efficient.

The other safeguard was that the Doctor checked the Drug book and cabinet on each of his fortnightly Clinics.

"TRUST ME, I'M AN AMBULANCE OFFICER."

I sat up in bed and automatically reached for the phone - the strident tone of its ring had woken me from a sound sleep - the type of sleep experienced only by the pure in heart with a clear conscience - as neither you nor I dear reader fall into that category, we must take it for granted.
My sound sleep was due to a long day, a cold winter's night, and the time of lowest resistance - 3am in the morning.

It was the Police Sergeant, "morning Mal, bloody cold eh! A car has crashed off the Pheasant Creek road, seems there's two fellows in it, don' know how badly but I'm on my way," came his report.
"Right Brian," I replied, shivering in my light pyjamas, "I'll see you there," and hung up, reached for a warm shirt and then my pressed white overalls I used for emergency night calls when time was of the essence. Grabbed my warm cap, hurried down stairs, into the Unit and off for Pheasant Creek until I came upon the Police car with its headlights illuminating the accident scene.

This was it alright. The broken fence and the fresh furrows in the red earth where the car had left the road, hit the water culvert, rolled and scrapped along the ground before coming to rest in the grazing paddock.

I got out into the clear morning air (boy, was it cold) I pulled my woollen cap over my ears and stumbled over the rough ground to the crashed car.

Brian (Sergeant Smart) indicated two figures, one sitting beside the car and leaning against it, the other sitting on the ground about 10 metres away - it was obvious that both were conscious and breathing, so I examined the man beside the car.

<u>Patient one</u>: conscious, coherent, pulse and breathing normal - normal that is for someone who had just crashed and rolled a car through a fence and was still alive, in other words they were a bit faster than average.
He had a probable fracture to his right arm, so I temporarily supported it in his shirt with a "you'll be right mate, I'll have you both in hospital in no time," as I quickly moved off to check the other chap who was still sitting over there looking at the ground.

<u>Patient two</u>: I walked over and crouched down beside him, "how are you mate?" I asked, placing my hand on his shoulder in a comforting manner.

"Up town," came the answer in a crooning tone. What have I got here I wondered!
"What happened?" I asked, trying another angle.
"Up town," came the same reply, with no change in his position still looking at the ground – my primary assessment was that he had suffered some degree of head injury, whether slight with some concussion / a fracture with concussion/ or of a

more serious nature involving actual injury to the brain and internal haemorrhage.

I placed my hand on his head to feel for any wetness or other injury, and went to speak to him, "I'm jus .... "

He looked up, and stared directly at me - a look of fright and alarm showed on his face and he moved to his hands and knees and shuffled backwards.

To say I was confounded was an understatement, I must have looked pretty astonished also, well, I always knew I was no oil painting, but I never thought I was ugly enough to frighten someone - it must be the old beanie cap over my ears!!
I snatched it off - that saved my pride a bit.

What a sight - there we were in an open paddock - I was crouched facing this chap who was on his hands and knees edging backwards away from me, and now I was moving towards him - then the famous words oft' repeated all over the world:-
"It's alright, YOU CAN TRUST ME, and I'M AN AMBULANCE OFFICER."

I ask you, who in their right mind, who saw two grown men on their hands and knees crawling around an open paddock at three o'clock in the morning, WOULD TRUST EITHER OF THEM!

Well, from his movements I at least assessed that he had no major injury to limbs or body, and I was able to calm him enough to coax him into the Ambulance and to transport him and his companion to the Mt. Morgan hospital.

He had suffered a severe concussion and was hospitalised for two weeks before being discharged fit and well.

Drought ravaged the district in 69-70 and accidents and treatments were subject to its dictates as illustrated by the next case:

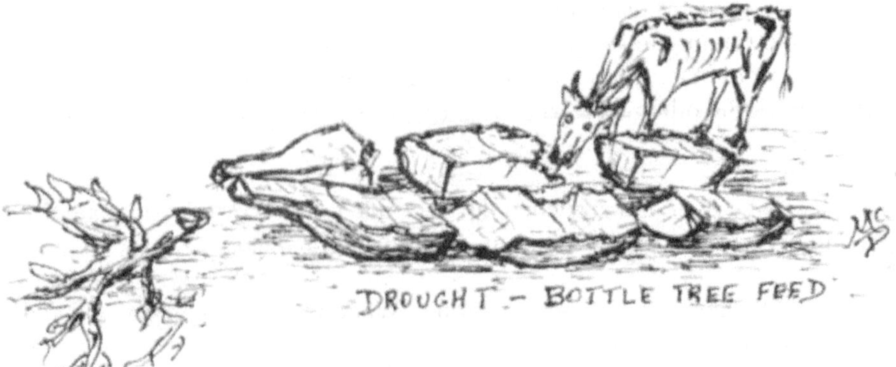

WHO'LL FEED THE STOCK - A Personal Tragedy.

In late 1969, Clyde Olsson a farmer from Pheasant Creek, rang the Casualty room bell at the Ambulance centre.

"Come in Clyde," I said, indicating the chair in the Casualty room, I noticed the clean rag around his left hand.

"What've you been up to?" I asked as I carefully untied the covering and disposed of it in the soiled dressings bin.
I washed my hands, and stepped back to inspect this injury.

" It's like this Malcolm, it was me jolly 'orse, I'd looped the bridle over me arm to undo the gate, when 'e threw 'is head back pulling the bridle, me finger caught on the piece of copper wire joining the reins," he replied, "silly thing to do."

I gently examined the finger, the loop of thin wire had neatly cut the tip off the first finger of his left hand, tearing through the finger nail and loosening the remaining segment.

I took a sterile bowl and two pair of forceps, and with sterile swabs and savlon solution (the dressing antiseptic at that date), carefully cleaned the surrounding area of the injury, then the wound and placed a sterile cover over it.

"Well Clyde we'll have to go to Mt. Morgan Hospital, you'll need a skin graft for that."

Clyde looked me straight in the eye, "**who'll feed and water the stock**?"

"Clyde, for the finger to heal properly, you'll need a skin graft, you'll only be in for a couple of days."

"Malcolm! the wife can't manage by herself, and the stock 'll die if I'm not there to do the heavy lifting, look, just clean it up and I'll come in each day."

Yes, I knew only too well what he was talking about, the district was still in drought, and farmers were struggling desperately to survive. Stock were being hand fed and water had to be carted to them in some cases.

If he was to stay and have daily dressings, I would require Doctors permission for the necessary treatment.
"Clyde, I'll ring the Doc and see what he has to say."

Dr. Mc Cosker realised the situation and advised an anti Tetanus injection, daily dressings of jellonet, antibiotic therapy of PVK 250mg.

"Right Clyde, let's at it, a shot of anti tetanus' first.

The District Health Inspector who also held Clinics at the Centre would leave a stock of injections for the Doctor to dispense when required.
"It'll sting a bit, then we'll dress your finger, and give you some tablets to take."

As there was no Doctor or hospital at Wowan, and the closest was 25 miles away at Mt Morgan, a recorded stock of drugs were held in my office, on behalf of the Doctor who would dispense same through me, and would check the supply against the record book every 2 weeks when he held his Clinic at the centre.

Every day Clyde would attend at the centre after he had cared for the stock, and I would clean and dress his wound and protect it with a leather finger stall.

As it progressed, I sometimes had him sit by the closed window, to give the healing wound some morning sun.

Needless to say Clyde's finger healed over a few weeks, it would have been much quicker if he had gone to hospital to possibly have a skin graft, and a lot less work for me, but at least he was able to care for his stock and keep his farm.

WORKLOAD and RELAXATION:

This was only one of the 2000 cases I attended for the 12 months, so the combination of cases, office administration, fundraising, centre cleaning etc., kept me busy and with the overall problems from the drought situation the job was pretty constant and demanding and one needed something to help one relax.

I gained this relaxation from an unexpected source - Vera Crawley had organised art classes in oil painting which were conducted on the Centre veranda every Saturday for a rental of 10 cents per student [top dollar stuff]. Vera asked me to join the class with the hope of encouraging other men to participate.

The instruction given by the Mt. Morgan artist taught us the basics of oil painting - all that was needed to get a start - the board or support, paints, brushes, charcoal sketch and application.

I enjoyed these lessons to the extent that I read a couple of books on oil painting and after a heavy day and on finishing the office bookwork about 10pm I might start to paint to relax and suddenly find it was 3am, but I was totally relaxed and mentally refreshed.

THE POOR COW:

1970 was still drought time for central Queensland and the local farmers and graziers had little to spend on bringing Veterinary surgeons up from Rockhampton. In truth the Vets from Rocky would not travel to Wowan because, it took more than time to obtain payment in the majority of cases.

Once I became known and respected for my ability as an Ambulance officer and assistant to the Doctor, then the locals reckoned I must be good enough for treating injuries to livestock.

An early client was Arthur McArthur; a small wiry man, weather beaten features, of indeterminate age, a human Popeye, quick short bursts of speech and full of fight. Arthur had been badly affected by the drought and was down to feeding his stock on peanut trash (the dry peanut plant leaves and branches after harvest of the nuts), he rang one Saturday morning.

" Mr. McDonald, Arthur McArthur here, I've got a cow that stepped in a crack in the ground and broke it's leg, can you come out and fix it ?"
"Arthur, you know I'm not a Vet and as far as I know if a cow has broken it's leg you may as well shoot her!"

" I can't afford to shoot her," he stated strongly," I rang the Butcher and he said he wouldn't buy 'er because she'd be too bruised, if you could only do something to allow the bruising to go away, then she could be slaughtered," he pleaded.

I knew what straits he was in, so I was persuaded, "alright I'll come out and have a look." Thanks, Mr. Mac."

I collected the gear I might need. 'Yes four rolls of plaster of Paris bandage, a couple of rolls of old cotton wool, mmmhh might be compound, better take some antibiotic dusting powder and two syringes of outdated procaine penicillin, that'll do.'

On arrival Arthur and his two sons took me out to the injured animal, she was in poor condition, standing favouring her front right leg, the ankle or fetlock area was swollen.

I looked around at the parched earth, and the wide cracks in the ground the radiated in all directions, "reckon you're lucky she didn't vanish altogether down one of them," I observed.

"Yeh! lost a truck the other day," he replied straight faced.

"Arthur you had better throw her, and have the lads hold her down."

Arthur's sons threw the cow very efficiently, one grasping her head and one horn and twisting, the other swinging on the tail, down she went, and down she stayed, with one sitting on her neck and one on her rump.

From a small disposable bowl filled it with antiseptic, using forceps, with swabs I cleaned the perforated area; I then dressed this with antibiotic powder and lint squares.

I applied the old cotton wool to the leg as padding for the plaster cast.

Arthur had returned with the fencing wire which I fashioned into a splint by bending it at 18 inches, I placed two plaster bandages in the water and when the first was useable applied it over the cotton wool for 18 inches from the top of the hoof up the leg, the wire splint was positioned over the first bandaging, and further plaster over this.

I then applied the other plaster bandage, then another. I examined my handiwork, not too bad for a mug.

"Now hold her head so I can give her this injection into her neck muscle," I commanded. I reckoned her size was worth two human doses, so gave her the two syringes of the outdated procaine penicillin.

" Well Arthur, that's about all I can do for her, but you must keep her still until that plaster cast sets, or our work is wasted."
"How long Mr. Mac ?"

"Sit on her until you get a tapping sound when you tap the cast with your knuckle, O'k ? I'll be off then."

" Thanks for all you've done Mr. Mac," said Arthur.
FOR ALL I'D DONE, what was that compared to the deprivation and hardship he and his family had been having for the past 12 months.

Well I didn't see Arthur to talk to for months and months, then one day I bumped into him at the Co-op store, "Arthur, how did that cow get on with the broken leg ?"

Arthur looked up and replied, "she's had a calf since then **but the fetlock is stiff !**" did I note a tone of accusation in his voice**?**

" Good," I said and walked on, only too pleased to know the beast had not died, Mmmugh, he's a survivor alright, he made the best of that setback and turned it to gain.

The next case was not due to drought just a case of animal welfare.

LOVE THAT DOG:

Mid afternoon and I was minding my own business, which is a change for an Ambulance officer, when Kev Cocks the Police constable, walked in from the Police station next door.

" How are you, Kev," I greeted him," things a bit quiet next door?" I enquired.

" Yer, I just finished a 'two foolscap pages' on that chap at Govigen a coupla days ago," Kev replied laconically.

The 'two foolscap pages' was the term for the length of the report police were required to write on any death which occurred outside a hospital.

" No it's me dog, he was in a fight with Carter's mongrel and got a good rip on the shoulder, I wondered if you would stitch it up for me," he asked.

Wonder what the other dog looks like then ? If Kev's dog got a 'good rip', I bet the other dog's booked in for a new fur coat.

This dog of Kevin's was as big as an Alsatian, of arrogant disposition, a jet black coat, so that the first thing you saw of him at night, was the sudden gleam of a full set of white fangs as big as Jaws, as he scared the shimoodle out of you, with a bark that lifted the hair on your neck, permanently.

“Wondered if you would stitch it up for me,” *rubbish*!, he knew that the Police and Ambulance helped each other out all the time, we depended on each other, so there was no risk that I would not help him this time -

UNLESS I WAS SCARED - NO, NOT ME - NOT MUCH.

" Right Kev, I'll do it, but I want the child that gets on the best with the dog to come with him, and to sit there with his hand on the dog's head while I stitch him up."

" No problem Mal, that's Terry, the dog loves him."

So Kevin turned up half an hour later with 7 year old son Terry, and the big ‘doggie.’

I lead them to the spare back room kept for this style of treatment, and indicated that the dog be placed up on the plastic, on the old wooden cas couch.

As I eyed off the 4 inch wound (10cm) in the dogs right shoulder, I instructed young Terry:

" Terry , the dogs been hurt and I'm going to sew up the cut he's got, but, every time I push the needle in it should hurt him, so I want you to talk to him all the time, and to keep patting him on the head, so he knows he is safe."

Well, I selected the suture, needle, forceps, swabs, antiseptic, and two pair of scissors.

I clipped the hair from around the wound, then cleaned the area and the wound.

I then commenced stitching, **one in**, **two in**, **three in**, good I've still got my hand, **f-o-u-r** - as the dog lifts it's head and looked back at me, then lay back again.

Yes, I'm sure that animals know when you are trying to help them, because I have never been bitten by any animal I was treating.

A couple more then a dab with a clean swab to finish the treatment, and the instruments into a basin for cleaning and sterilisation before storing in the "Vet" cupboard.

All's well that ends well, but when Kev saw me a week later and said, " ah Mal, what about takin' those stitches out?" He loved to have a crack.

I replied most courteously, "Kev, old chap, you may remove the stitches yourself," or words to that effect.

As you have now concluded, Ambulance and Police officers in country areas, share many experiences.

THE EYES SAID IT ALL.

The inland or outback can be lonely in more ways than one.

I remember receiving a call from a traveller who had come across a single car accident on the lonely road between Biloela and Wowan. There was only the car smashed into the trunk of a large tree beside the road with the injured driver still in the vehicle.

The traveller had to leave the injured man to drive to the nearest dwelling or telephone to ring the Ambulance.
"There's a bloke unconscious in a car back along the road to Biloela," came tumbling out of the phone, a gasp for breath, then, "he ran off the road and hit a tree," completed the statement.

"Where are you now? and how far back was the accident ?" I asked.
"Where am I" I heard him ask. "I'm at Vimy, and I suppose the accident was about 12 miles (20K) back," he replied.

When I tried to get more accurate directions, it became obvious that the traveller was not familiar with the area and really was not sure just how far away the accident site was.
Information from a stranger can be very inaccurate and could be many miles out because the person is most concerned to get help to the injured and they don't think to look at their speedo until they are somewhere down the track.

As this had the probability of serious injury, and there was already a time factor from impact to reporting the accident, I quickly made ready to leave.
I called Val, made a quick report on the situation, asked her to ring Biloela Centre and to inform them fully as the accident might well be close to their end of the road.

I drove off in emergency mode and kept driving until I came upon the lone vehicle, bonnet smashed into the tree beside the road.
A quiet peaceful scene, cattle grazing in the paddock nearby, a few parrots picking seeds from the road verge and in the distance a scroll of trees marking the creek.
I slowed and pulled off the road careful to control braking in the loose gravel of the roadside, and stopped facing the crashed vehicle.

I could see the injured driver still sitting behind the wheel head tilted to one side.
'Could be unconscious' I thought and hoped, you don't think 'fatal,' you stay positive ready to act.
I grabbed my kit from beside the seat, scrambled out and hurried around to the driver's side of the crashed vehicle.
As I approached I was noting every detail to assist in my diagnosis of my patient.

His head was tilted to the left but facing slightly to the to the right so that I could see his eyes were open, 'good should be conscious,' a couple of steps closer and to could see the clearness of his eyes, 'beaut- definitely alive and conscious.'

"You'll be right mate," I said loud and clear to establish contact and give reassurance. He'd been out here for the past hour at the very least from when the traveller had first came upon the accident.

He didn't say anything, but I saw his eyes follow me as I moved closer to the door and as I looked in through the open driver's window.

"I'll look after you," I said, "where are you hurt?" I continued.

His clear blue eyes looked alertly into mine, but he did not answer.

In the emergency situations your adrenalin is pouring out and your mind is intently and rapidly examining every piece of information presented, be it from sight, smell, hearing or touch, and this information is tabled against previous knowledge and experience.
Smell had given me the information of engine smell of oil and machinery but no petrol or heat, nor was there any smell of blood or vomit.
The touch of my hand on his right shoulder told me the body was warm, it was a clear sunny day.

My eyes told me that his skin colour was normal, he had no injuries to his face nor to his shoulders, his eyes were clear and alert, he was aware because his eyes were always looking into mine when I looked back into his face after each look away to check for other info.
My ears were not giving any answers, breathing not noisy, but no answers to my greeting or questions – 'could he be dumb?'

"How are you mate, have you any pain?" I tried again.
He looked into my eyes but no answer.

WHAT IS IT, I asked myself – my mind raced over the information my senses were providing – conscious-breathing quietly- no blood – eyes alert- no voice !!
EYES ALERT – EYES SPEAKING TO ME – eyes saying – "I KNOW THERE IS NO HOPE" they despaired.
OH HELL, the answer shouted at me – fractured cervical spine with severe damage to the spinal cord with a loss of feeling and movement below the fracture.

This was my first severe spinal case of quadriplegia, and it was now very lonely beside that country road.

I quietly said, "I'll look after you mate, I'll just get some things from the ambulance," but the eyes did not respond with sign of thanks, just the clear alert stare with the underlying message of despair.

I returned and pinned a folded towel firmly around his neck as support.

Then I heard the sound of an approaching car, it was the Biloela Ambulance.

I quickly gave a full report to the Biloela Ambulance officer and we discussed how to extricate the patient from the car to a stretcher.
Garth and I carefully supported and lifted the patient from the car onto a blanketed stretcher beside us. We immobilised our patient's head and neck with appropriate sandbags, adjusted the blanket, and carefully secured him to the stretcher.

We had decided that Garth would transport the patient to Biloela Hospital as this was the closest Medical care, so as soon as the patient was loaded we each drove off in opposite directions, back to our respective towns and Centres to be available for the next emergency or call for assistance.

It was a long time before I lost the vision of those eyes looking into mine, so clear, so alert but silent, yet 'those eyes said it all.'

WHY ME ?

There was no Care Flight - there was no SES – but there was RAIN.

There had been some very heavy rain from a number of storms as well as intermittent showers over the past few days, so that the country was soaked and the creeks running.

I received the phone call from the Overseer of a station outside Wowan on the other side of a tributary of the Dawson, about eight-thirty one evening.

" I've got a young feller working for me who was a bit off today and he's not getting any better, and now he says he's got a pain in his side, with the creek up and this pain we're a bit worried, what do'ya reckon ?"

'What do I reckon?', well I was 'reckoning' a number of things, (how high was the creek), what were the other signs and symptoms ? (how high was the creek), how long had he been ill ? (how high was the creek), how old ? (how high was the creek), and the big one - had he had his appendix removed ?

I asked all those questions and a couple more. I then rang the Doctor at Mt. Morgan.

" Doc, I've got a 20 year old male, who complained this morning of nausea with slight stomach pain. The pain has localised to the right side and he feels worse, the creek is up and his boss is concerned as to whether he should be in hospital," I reported, and waited for the questions.

" No, he has not had his appendix removed, no, he has not had any falls from a horse or accidents to cause an internal injury or muscle strain - sorry I missed constipation, don't know - I'll check on the fever too, be back to you shortly."

I rang the station and checked the questions Doctor required answered, then rang him back.

" He hasn't had a bowel motion today, (although that was not the question I had heard asked of the patient by his boss) and he might be a bit warm, and yes they say he has gradually worsened through the day and is still 'going down'," I reported.

"By that report we can't take any chances, he'll have to come in to the hospital for examination and observation at the least, and immediate surgery if required," came the Doctor's decision, " and tell them he is not to have anything to eat or drink, and to list what he has had for the last four hours."

" Righto we'll start into it, but it could be a while before we get him in to you, the creeks running a banker I'm told and until we reach the creek we won't know how bad things are," I replied.

I rang the station and informed the station Overseer of the Doctor's decision and his instructions, then asked the state of the creek crossing.

He told me that one of the station hands had just returned from checking the road, and had reported the creek to be running a banker, flowing fast and the rain continuing.

" Good enough," I replied resignedly," I want you to pack the lad's gear, but leave a change of clothes separate in a plastic bag, make him comfortable in your car, and to bring ropes and torches with you to the crossing, we'll be leaving in about 15 minutes, oh! and don't forget a couple of strong station hands," I advised.

I contacted the Police Sergeant and informed him of the situation, and that it was too risky to leave the patient, that he had to come into the hospital in case a operation was required.

Sergeant Brian Smart said," O'k, but it could be a 'bit risky' for us too before the night's out, I'll get onto Kev straight away."

I thanked him then prepared for the trip, spare torch, coil of rescue rope, raincoat and hat, Val came down with a flask of coffee and some sandwiches.

Well that's about it, with a good-bye to the family and my sister who was down for a couple of weeks, I set off for the creek crossing and whatever it had to offer, it was well after nine pm by this.

When I arrived at the crossing I was a bit surprised to say the least, I had expected a flooded creek crossing that might be negotiated by throwing ropes across or whatever and pulling or assisting someone across.

What I saw before me in the light from the Ambulance unit, was a stretch of dirty, brown, angry water, 25 metres wide, with a few metres of quiet water each side.

' Bloody hell!' and I thought this was going to be a simple flooded creek transfer, a bit of hard work, a bit of discomfort, a bit of danger for spice, **but NOT THIS.**

The area of the actual crossing and the other bank was clear of trees, but the flooded creek had broached the banks and reached into the tree growth on this side.

This was going to be a real problem.

Kevin the Police Constable arrived with a couple of helpers, and shortly after the Overseer with the patient and two station hands pulled up on the other side of the creek.

Kev had one look, turned to me and drawled dryly," could be a bit tricky Mal, could be a bit tricky."

We called questions and answers across to each party, and passed some suggestions on how the river, (yes it was better than a creek now), could be crossed, but none of them were very convincing.

Kev walked into the backwater at the road crossing, but it was up to his chest after a few metres so it ruled out trying to drive a truck over.

The Overseer had said it was too deep, but it had to be tested and not taken for granted.

On the other side a strong looking young station hand stripped down to his shorts and waded in, then started swimming, but was washed down about fifty metres until he grabbed a tree to save himself going further.
This was pretty useless even if he had reached us, because he brought nothing with him and caused us to waste at least thirty minutes, struggling through the scrub, making numerous attempts to throw a rope to him, then finally tying one end to a piece of dead wood, throwing it out and floating it down to him.

We then tried to throw the rope across the water by attaching a rock to the end and swinging it around as in casting a fishing line, but we didn't do any good, it hardly reached halfway.

Back to the crossing and talk it over, nothing very illuminating came from that, except that the Doctor be contacted and informed of the situation.

I radioed the Centre and asked Val to ring the Doctor and inform him of our problem, and ask for any suggestions.

The radio squawked into life," Wowan control to Wowan car 1," I answered and Val gave the message," Doctor said that if the patient has not improved then he should be transported to hospital, as it is too big a risk to leave him."

I knew the answer but I called the question to the Overseer, his reply floated clearly over the water," no change, just as bad, if not worse."

'Well that's that, finger out and do something' I mused to myself.

Another huddle, and we decided that some stronger rope should be obtained, joined to the lighter rope we had with us, so that the light rope could be attached to a person who would walk out as far as he could, then swim for the other side.

The light rope was for two actions, one to pull the person back to safety if the current sweep him downstream too fast, or secondly to pull the heavier rope across after he reached the other side, as a life line for helpers and the patient.

It was also decided that the one to go across should be someone who could examine the patient and diagnose his condition - now who would that be ?, no prize for second, - ' **WHY ME** ' ? yes it was logical.

I again radioed Val and asked her to get some strong rope from the Sergeant and to bring it out to us, I didn't tell her why.

Val arrived about thirty minutes later with the rope and a few packets of biscuits for the men, it was now about one am.
[We had an arrangement with a couple of the Ladies Committee members, Mrs. Ford and Mrs. Burgraff, both widows, who would either come to the Centre during the night, or Val would drop off the children to them during the day, at short notice.]

We joined the ropes, and tied a loop with a bowline, and I stripped down to my underpants.

There was much comment as to my general physique, and to how I'd go broke as a strip tease artist.

I waded into the water and the chaps eased the line out after me - the water reached my waist and pulled at my legs, it was damn cold at this hour of the night.
I waded further and the current was stronger with the depth of water - I was leaning into the current and struggling to keep my footing - I inched my way further - the water up to my armpits.

GLUG - my legs were swept from under me - head under the current - mouthful of water - strike out freestyle - I could feel the current carrying me downstream - the rope tightened around my chest and I was pulled backwards - it's not nice against the current - the water forced itself up my nose and into my eyes before I rolled onto my side; I was dragged back to the bank like a stunned mullet, because Kev could see that the current was too strong to allow a landing, especially with the rope dragging behind me.

Another council of war, this was interrupted by the Police car radio, it was the Sergeant, he had rung around and had found someone with an aluminium dingy and had 'requested' the owner to take it to us, Brian said he should be arriving shortly.

This was good news, for we really had tried everything we could, and were at a loss as to what we could try next.

Well the rest was so easy in comparison - the boat arrived and was unloaded - the rope was attached to the stern - Kev and I boarded and took a oar each –

the chaps gave the boat a mighty heave forward - we strained at the oars, and gave it a 'dozen' - the light boat skimmed over the rushing water.

We landed, loaded our patient, retied the rope to the bow, gave a yell to the mob on the other side, a jerk forward, and we were pulled back across the river.

I transported my patient to the highway then on to Mt. Morgan hospital, I have to admit that the road vanished from sight a couple of times, because I had worked a normal day before this 16 hour stint, but we reached the hospital safely and I had a cup of coffee and drove back to Wowan and bed at last.

Another case completed all in the days (and nights) work for an Ambulance family at a one man Centre, but then what else would you expect ?

Next time I called in to Rocky centre the chaps complained about us being noisy on the radio and disturbing them all night, as I said, *what else would you expect.*

TRAINING BEFORE 1970:

Training within the Ambulance Service in Queensland before 1970, was totally dependent on Committees and the Superintendent and the industry of the officer.

The text books used by the C.A.T.B. after 1892 were manuals from the Royal Army Medical Corps, followed by the British Red Cross Society First Aid manual after 1912, the Warwick and Tunstall's Advanced Ambulance Handbook.

The St John Home Nursing and Home Hygiene manuals were also used in later years as basic text books for entry to the Q.A.T.B. , and the St John First Aid handbook was used by the Ambulance Service to teach First Aid to the community and organisations.

As the Superintendent was the technical adviser to the Committee, he was responsible for the level of training at that centre.

In a few instances a Committee might dictate the level of training but this was the result of the Superintendents inability to educate the Committee on the current status of Pre-hospital Care and the needs of the community. This reflected on the level of knowledge of that Superintendent.

The dedication and enthusiasm of the Bearer in the early days was exactly similar to that of our dedicated officers of today, for in my appointments to various centres throughout Queensland, I have found text books of a very high standard for their day, now dusty and put away.

Books ranging from 'Gray's Anatomy 1880'; 'Medicology' by Joseph Richardson Professor of Hygiene, University of Pennsylvania 1908 edition; 'Manual of Splints and Appliances' reproduced by permission of the United States Army, issued by the British Red Cross society 1917; Murrell's 'What to do in cases of Poisoning'; Warwick and Tunstall's 'First Aid to the Injured and Sick', an Advanced Ambulance Handbook.

Treatments certainly have changed for some conditions, "Wasp stings" being a good example, as can be shown by the treatment administered for a Wasp sting in the early part of that century:-

Treatment:- 1. Make the patient lie down and give stimulants freely.
Brandy, whisky and champagne are useful.
If swallowing impossible, inject with an enema apparatus, into the rectum.

Thankfully medical treatments have progressed in this area – well, have certainly improved.

On the front shelf were copies of Sears, Anatomy and Physiology for Nurses; Miller and Keane Encyclopaedia and Dictionary of Medicine and Nursing etc.

I mentioned in a previous chapter how Dr Lester demonstrated on one of his own staff, (who was undoubtedly willing, but unconscious at the time), the technique for maintaining an airway, for my edification.

In those early years the larger provincial centres such as Cairns, Townsville and Rockhampton under Superintendents Hogan, McIntosh and Daniel organised staff training lectures.

This continued into the early 60's under Superintendents like Tom Briggs who organised regular lectures for the Cairns staff, presented by local Doctors, and attended all lectures himself.

I clearly remember sitting beside him one night when the Lecturer paused and Supt Briggs asked, "Doctor why should we use splints for fractured legs, wouldn't padding between the legs and a few broad bandages be quicker, and just as good?"

I was astounded, Tom Briggs was the best in Queensland, he was the hero of the Aerial Ambulance, he should know the answer, even I as a young honorary, knew why splints were used.

Thinking about it later I realised that Tom Briggs certainly knew the answer and more, but he also knew that staff who didn't know, would not ask in case others thought they were stupid, so Tom, with his high reputation at risk, asked on their behalf.
This too was a lesson for me, and I have asked many questions over the years, not because I didn't know the answer, but on behalf of others.

About this time, in the late 50's Brisbane centre commenced staff lectures in earnest and these continued with the assistance of local Doctors and Medical specialists, one of the most noted being Dr Ken Jamieson.

Late one night at Julia Creek, I transported a patient to Dr Duggan's surgery, and attended with the patient in case the Doctor required assistance.
Dr Duggan examined the patient, speaking aloud as he proceeded, "now examine each quadrant, applying careful, steady pressure, the patient will quickly alert you to any tenderness, whether by a guarding of that part, by a grimace of pain, or vocally."

The patient raised his head slightly and asked, "WHAT'S THAT DOC?"
It may sound familiar, but it was asked.

Arthur Duggan smiled at the patient, "It's alright Charlie, lie back, I'm explaining a few things to the Ambulance Bearer," and continued, "If there is no pain on gentle pressure, you can release that pressure suddenly checking for rebound tenderness etc."

Thus I received patient care training at odd hours and in different circumstances such as when I donated blood, even then Doc Duggan explained each step, (although I could have done without it at that time), but training I got, and my skills improved.

When I took my first annual leave from Julia Creek, I was hospitalised with Hepatitis in Cairns.
Dr Wilson and I had some discussions on Emergency situations and he loaned me a copy of "Pye's Surgical Handicraft" which I studied assiduously over those weeks of convalescence. I absorbed the information with supporting references and this formed the basis for my future pre-hospital care and emergency procedures.

At Rockhampton Doctors Learmonth, O'Duffy, McClymont, Agnew, Everingham and the various Hospital Casualty department Doctors all instructed us in one way or another.
We in turn instructed lay people in First aid, and did this as a community service, whereas today, all First aid instructors are paid to conduct classes.

Officers would discuss cases when they returned to centre, and suggestions would be offered as assistance, or as an improvement in patient care.

Just after I took up my position as Driver bearer at Rocky, Terry Noonan demonstrated the false capeline head bandage, which was applied more quickly than the full capeline, an important feature in the emergency situation, thus officers taught each other.

These discussions also gave support to officers who returned from fatal or distressing cases, and were suffering an emotional reaction.

Unfortunately at some Brisbane stations in 1991, when officers return to station there is little discussion, because the TV is showing some mind warping program and anyone who speaks is immediately shushed by the mediocre officers who are listening and completing reports at the same time, or the TV volume is increased.

To overcome this lack of peer support, the service now has trained staff Counsellors available and further professional staff if required.

I also attended 'night school' (as it was called then), at the Rockhampton Technical College, enrolling in the course "Practical Bookkeeping and Business Studies", which covered general Office procedures from ordering goods, receipting and banking monies, record keeping and basic accounting.

This self training was practised by the dedicated officers.

Over some years the Q.A.T.B. discussed proposals for a Training School for Ambulance officers, but had done nothing further, even though the discussions were at the level where officers from interstate had been invited to participate.

The NSW Ambulance service commenced a training School for its officers in 1968, and invited representatives from Queensland to attend.

1970 WAS ALSO THE 150 ANNIVERSARY OF WOWAN CENTRE:

Of course the 'Super' was tasked with the organisation of the celebrations:-

The Centenary Parade and unveiling of the Pioneer Plinth was a major event before the Centenary Ball that night.

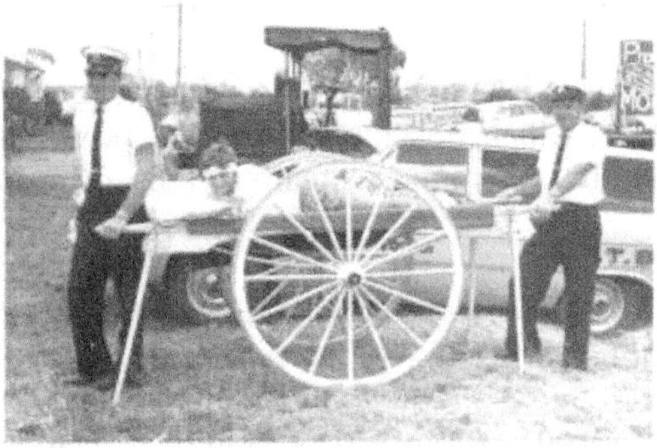

Mick Davis and J. Cook & Ashford Litter.

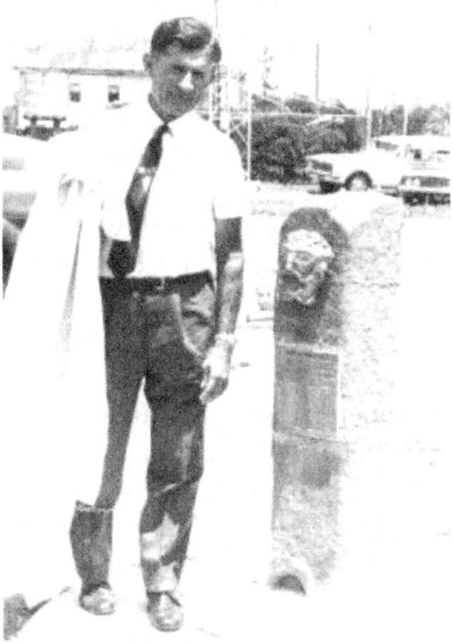

Shire Chair unveils Pioneer Plinth, sculptured by Malcolm McDonald.

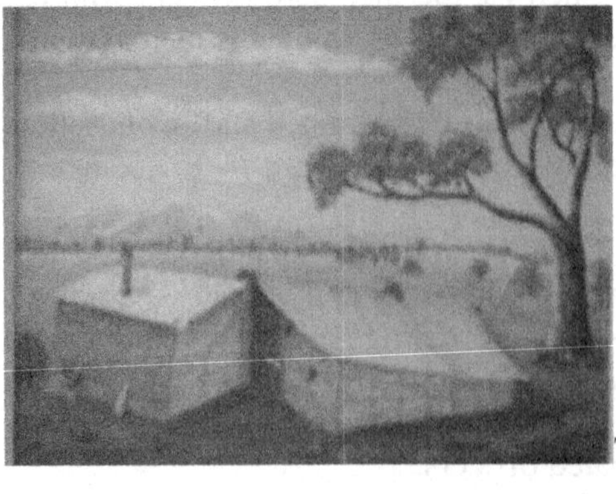

Temporary Wowan sub Centre 1917

QATB STATE TRAINING SCHOOL – 1970.

HOW MUCH SAFER - HOW MUCH EASIER - WHY NOT?

In 1970 Queensland followed NSWs and organised the first Q.A.T.B. State Training School and conducted Stage 1 Course 1for Superintendents.
The curriculum included subjects on:- anatomy and physiology, emergency and pre-hospital care procedures, rescue and extrication, cannulation and infusion, IV and IM injections. Sadly this was as far as these procedures ventured – the Medical hierarchy of the time controlled any further progress.
The course ran for two weeks, day and evenings, with a further one week course on management and administration, conducted by the Australian Institute of Management.

As QATB Wowan did not have spare monies, I took holidays so I could attend the Training School.

Stage 1, Course 1 provided subjects of:-

1. ADMINISTRATION: basic management, planning and human resource management skills. [Institute of Management]

Management conducted by the Australian Institute of Management was one of the most important segments of Stage 1for me. [I already practiced the advanced skills of no touch techniques and injections, and had experience of dispensing medications at Wowan].

We were taught 'The Management Process' and more:-
Types of Leadership - Decision making and Direction and ensuring they are understood - Motivation and needs of the individual = self esteem/ achievement/ reward/ security/ greed/ money and so on.

Budgeting = traditional/actual/projected; the target audience; control.
I developed my own budget strategy, *ie*, finance to be conservative on income estimates with a buffer for emergencies, to be practical on expenditure, any surplus finance directed to identified projects/expansion – must be a flexibility to change direction if any unanticipated difficulty arose, ie reviews and adjust pathway when necessary.
One could even develop a strategy for most initiatives using these principles.

2. ADVANCED LIFE SUPPORT skills and techniques:
   Pseudo certification of skills for :-
   - casualty room procedures. This addressed no touch techniques ; sterilisation of equipment and instruments; wounds and haemorrhage.
   - childbirth; injections and cannulation, etc by Registered Nurse Doig, triple certificate followed by attendance at BGH:-

Casualty; Maternity; Cardiac; Pathology; Intensive Care and Out Patient Departments.

- Advanced Life Support techniques by Medical Officers & Training Officer Cliff Coddington.

All lectures concluded with questions by the Medical Officer so that any follow-up could be attended to by the Training Officer.

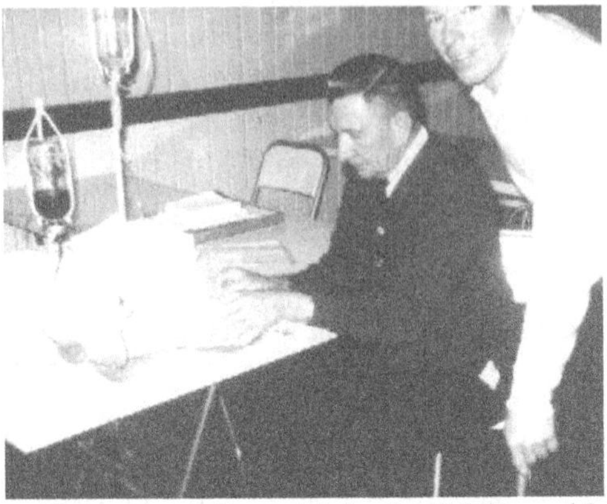

Supt. Tom Briggs and Supt. Malcolm McDonald at Stage 1 Training School.

I must make pertinent observations at this point :-

1. This training was opposed by certain people within the Service, on the principle that Superintendents were well experienced, and on the Industrial front there was no increase in wages to attend.

2. The management component by the Australian Institute of Management was a vital need for Superintendents who had received no formal training, but this excellent course was dropped because of costs? How negative.

3. Management subjects were never included in later years, much to the long term cost of the Service and its officers.

Because of this opposition by the Union in general, and by a number of Superintendents due to fear of the unknown, the QATB State Council had difficulty in obtaining numbers for Course 1.

I made sure I attended, I took holidays from Wowan Centre, [because they could not really afford to 'give' me three weeks], the Centre gave me the use of a sedan to travel and paid any other costs, so I was able to attend.

The Institute of Ambulance Officers (Aust.) had their inaugural meeting in Canberra in 1973, and moved to develop Australian standards of Pre-hospital care, and a standard of education and training for ambulance officers.
The Institute organised workshops at Monash University in 1974, with

representatives from:- the Royal colleges of Surgeons, Medicine, Nursing, Anaesthetists, etc, Departments of health and Education, Ambulance Authorities, and from the I.A.O. (Aust).

This group developed the syllabus of knowledge and skills required for a qualified Ambulance officer as a member of the Health team.
This Syllabus was the reference for the National Education Committee, a Standing Committee of the I.A.O. (Aust) to further develop a curriculum of 12 then 17 units for the training of Ambulance officers throughout Australia.

Again there was Industrial opposition to increased training, on the pretext of wage increases for skills, whereas the main opposition originated from the fear of pass or fail structured training.

The Victorian Ambulance service used the Institutes curriculum as the base requirements for their Certificate in Applied Science, (Ambulance).

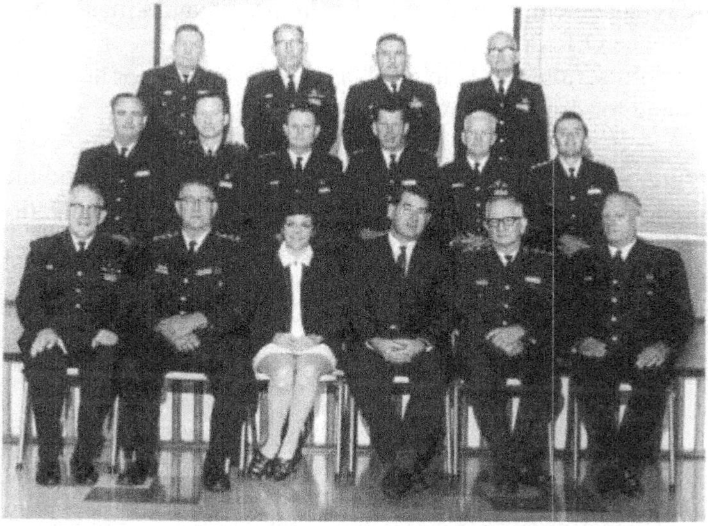

Stage 1, Course 1, QATB State Council Training School – July 1970.
Top: Supt. Tom Briggs; O.I.C. G. Brittain; Sen. Off. A. Butcher; D/Supt. Patrick. 2nd row: D/Supt. M. Meacham; Supt. Bert Toogood; Supt. Jack Stibbs; Supt. Malcolm McDonald; S. Off. A. Doeberitz; Supt. Brian Moore
Front: Supt. Eric Bannerman; Supt. Fred Leader; 3rd Cert. RN Doig; CTO Cliff Coddington; Supt. Gordon Stuart; Supt. Reg Bartels.

The biggest mistake the State Council made in all their years was to remove the Management segment from Training Courses for Superintendents – the QATB paid dearly for this especially in 1991
I had, and used, my papers and notes on this Management Course up to 2001.

There was opposition to Superintendents attending this introductory Course which was tailored especially for them – a 'letter' was circulated stating this opposition.

The State Council found it hard to get enough Superintendents to attend, in fact they allowed two Deputies and a Senior Bearer to make up numbers.
Though the letter was not signed it was believed it was circulated by the Secretary of the Superintendents Association.

§To risk simplification – self study, experience with trauma cases from scene to Hospital - timeframe and the observation of treatments/procedures administered by Doctors in Casualty, [including 'cut down' when venous collapse denied access for infusion], convinced me that:- damage to vital internal organs from reduced blood volume in cases of trauma could be averted either partly or completely by the maintenance of circulating blood volume through the intervention at scene by supplying fluid replacement, *ie* intravenous cannulation and infusion by the qualified Ambulance Officer.
This would maintain serious cases in a salvageable condition or at the least make available the venue for drug therapy etc.

As a regular regime at Wowan Centre Casualty I dispensed drugs and medication [either from stock or Chemist delivery via bus] and administered injections on the Doctors instruction.
So from personal experience I was aware of the controls and abilities required for this.

EDUCATION and TRAINING IS THE KEY.

It was obvious to me that the education and training of Ambulance officers was of the utmost importance to provide an acceptable level of pre-hospital care to the community.

It was obvious because :-

- *I had studied enough and had been assisted by local medicos to realise my shortcomings and the needs of the patient.*
- *When you had administered basic treatments in the field, then, on arrival at surgery or hospital casualty, in the first few minutes you witnessed a set of emergency procedures being followed which were common for all trauma cases.*
- *Text book after text book on pre-hospital emergency care preached the same message of necessary procedures.*
- *So, when we went to Brisbane on one of the few occasions, I had decided to pay a visit to the Medical School of Anatomy at the University to see what I could learn from any of their exhibits.*
- *In all innocence I presented myself at the Queensland University Medical School of Anatomy and asked if I might speak with the Head of the School - I received the rather patronising questions as to why I wished to see ANYONE?, who was I?, why did I want to see the Anatomy section ?, etc. etc. and finally the rather curt dismissal.*

I had maintained my composure throughout the questioning and in my answers as I believed that I could learn something which would give me a better understanding of the body and thus assist me in my diagnosis and treatment of various injuries, but on this cool dismissal I seethed with indignation for not having been taken seriously.
The adrenalin was pumping, my mind was in overdrive - I examined this - I rejected that - I re-examined this and spat out that - finally I calmed to a simmering aggression.

- STOP, let's look at this –
- do I really want to see what the School has to offer –
- do I really believe that it will assist me in understanding injuries-
- do I really believe that this knowledge will benefit my patients –

The answer to all of these came out as a definite YES - ***so do something.***

Do I know anyone who can HELP ?, is there someone who could 'step over' the self imposed gatekeepers.
Normally I would not ask anyone to help me personally, I generally did things for myself because I found it difficult to ask someone for a personal favour and I certainly did not indulge in using family friends to my own advantage, BUT, *this was different, this was for knowledge to assist me in my job of patient care.*

The inspiration came to me - Claude Mann, Dr. Claude Mann, he was a Specialist on Wickham Terrace, his father had been a benefactor of the Queensland University and I thought Claude might be on the Senate or something, anyway as an old family friend, [even though I had not seen him for many years], he would at least advise me.
I rang him up at his rooms.

After identifying myself to his receptionist, I was put through and Claude answered with a friendly greeting.
After we had exchanged family news and what I was doing in the Ambulance Service, I informed him of my unsuccessful visit to the Uni and why I wanted to visit the School of Anatomy etc.
Claude listened, asked some pertinent questions, then said, "I'll see what I can do, give me 24 hours, then ring me at 7am at home and I'll inform you of results," I thanked him and rang off.

I dutifully rang the morning after the next day at 7am and Claude answered, " right Malcolm, go to the school of Anatomy, ask for Mr......, tell him I sent you and he will take you through, then, when you have finished there go to the Medical School at Herston, ask for Mr........., tell him I sent you and he will take you through there."
I thanked him in a bit of a daze at my good fortune, and hung up.

I was out at the University by 9am, and my reception could not have been different. On identifying myself and my 'sponsor' I was received as a special visitor and taken throughout the dissection rooms and the preserving rooms and had all explained in a full and interesting manner, as it turned out, the visit was enlightening but not as educational as I had hoped.

I then attended at the Medical school at Herston, I identified myself and asked for Mr.........
This gentleman arrived and I again identified myself and that Dr. Claude Mann had made the arrangements, I was received with a reserved, courteous manner, and shown in to the Specimen area, *oh what a sight*, rows of jars of different sizes with all types of body specimens, clearly labelled, but with the history of the case/injury/disease, *it was a treasure trove of knowledge.*

As the curator assessed my motives and saw my sincerity his manner thawed and his attitude changed to one of openness and assistance, and shortly he left me unattended to study as long as I wished.

What a wonderful experience, I could not help but learn, I had the visual sample, the written case history, the established diagnosis of the injury/condition, and also access to a slide to examine under the microscope - hours later I left sated –
I could not hold any more - but the vision was recalled when I later studied the relevant text book.

I know that this one intense visit was a great benefit to all my future patients, for I was able to make a better diagnosis of my patient's injuries or condition, because I could understand more fully the way the body was affected, and how this in turn affected the patient, and thus how the patients felt and would react.

A few years later after the QATB had opened the Ambulance Training School I told the Chief Training Officer Rob Mc Dermott about the value in visualising injuries and conditions. He was able to obtain permission and to make arrangements for certain classes to attend at the Herston Medical School for a session.

Thus, the consideration of one man, in an eminent position, whose time was most valuable, gave benefit indirectly to many patients throughout Queensland.

DR. GARY R. MARTIN
M.B., B.S. (QLD.)

ASHMORE SHOPPING PLAZA
ASHMORE, Q., 4215
Phone: (075) 39 1677

November 29, 1979

Ambulance Board of Queensland

Dear Sir/Sirs,

I worked with Mr. Malcolm McDonald for three years when he was stationed at Wowan.

I was Medical Superintendent of Mt. Morgan Hospital, and worked in close association with him.

I found his degree of skill and competence were above the expected level for an Ambulance bearer and was able to rely on his verbal assessment of a patient's condition and was able to give directions over the telephone knowing that he could competently carry out my orders.

He was able to save me many valuable hours by treating patients with drugs which I was able to order from a special selection I had arranged at Wowan and tide patients over until the next day.

He was extremely interested in his patient's condition and particularly keen to follow up their medical care.

He often assisted me with critical cases such as fractures, setting up intravenous infussions and general care of unconscious patients. He was always keen to assist in minor surgical procedures.

I have always found him to be relied on to perform under all circumstances no matter how demanding and hereby recommend him for any position requiring competence, drive and foresight.

Yours sincerely,

Dr. G. R. Martin

QATB MALENY.

1972 appointment to Maleny placed me closer to the decision making and availability to attend State meetings – it also gave me space to gain experience in diplomacy and managing resources.
Inaugural meeting of the Institute of Ambulance Officers (Aust.) held in Canberra 1973 – McDonald a Founder Member

Maleny was a testing ground with a totally unresponsive Chairman and it was only due to a general request by Commissioner Self to inspect Centres of various status/employees that my Centre was fully inspected and I received a most complementary report which assisted my later appointment to Gatton.

TO TAKE THE INITIATIVE.

I made the decision that trauma patients in the pre-hospital situation should be given the benefit of the appropriate treatment and procedure to replace/maintain blood volume when indicated.

THE INITIATIVE WAS to show that Ambulance officers could be educated and trained to deliver the required level of Pre-hospital Emergency patient care which gave the optimum benefit for the recovery of injured or ill patients *ie management of the airway and cannulation at scene* for :- replacement of fluids/ drug therapy/ cannula in situ before vein collapse.

THE STRATEGY was to have it proven before it could be stopped.

THE HIGHLIGHTS would be the achievements along the way to gain the final gaol, of qualified Ambulance Officers administering Advanced Life Support procedures to patients.

A number of people held the opinion that Ambulance officers had a poor education and were not capable of learning.

I believed that a high percentage of the average ambulance officer of the 1970/80 era could be educated and trained.
The trick was THE WAY IN WHICH THE EDUCATION WAS PROVIDED

The second concern was what would happen to officers who did not, could not, pass the training programme as set out – there was no actual difficulty in meeting this need, the problem was more perceived than actual.

For the Ambulance officer to advance past the administration of Advanced First-aid was a problem BUT the real problem was how to overcome the prejudice and opposition by certain parties :-

1. Members of the Medical profession who were entrenched in the Health Department, the Educational faculties and in Politics, used arguments like: 'but Queensland is different to NSWs or Seattle." or "but Queensland has different problems."

My comment was "people bleed the same everywhere."
The Victoria Ambulance was a total NO! NO! as there was extreme derision by a Queensland Anaesthetist to anything the Victorian anaesthetist DR. Kamasoris proposed, developed, published or invented.
Their common remarks, "it's better to do nothing than to do harm" or " a little knowledge can be a dangerous thing."
Another favourite went something like "Advanced procedures are dangerous in untrained hands." **But all officers would be trained**.

This inferred that Ambulance officers could kill a patient by attempting Advanced procedures and this was used to great effect by this Doctor when speaking with Health and Community officials.
Of course those non-medical persons ran scared of future liability because they were aware that even 'trained and qualified Medical Officers also had fatalities with their procedures.'

2. The Nursing profession at that time were jealous of Ambulance officers administering techniques denied them.
3. Ambulance officers without an education above Scholarship were fearful of their ability to study and pass an examination.
4. The Union held the basic concept of money first, then training – the negative norm.

Superintendent Reg Bartels said that Brisbane A/Os were too dumb and Medical matters were for Doctors. Training Officer Bob McDermott in his reply to the IAO(Aust) syllabus for qualified Ambulance Officers, that it would result in an 100 % fail. The extreme example he gave re spontaneous pneumothorax was a smoke screen, this was his mentor talking.

Some Doctors took positions within the QATB structure to maintain Medico / Health Dept control. Possibly as Department policy.
Dr. Don Watson maintained the Health Department policy, but was more open to the needs of the patient and recognised genuine commitment to patient care.

There would be some wins and some losses and the need for the employment of some very careful strategies.

1972? – QATB State Conference Rockhampton – QATB Brisbane Chair Jim Arkell proposed St. John First Aid certificate be retained and QATB First aid certificate not be issued.

Supt. Mc Donald believed this to be unjust and spoke against the motion with vigour and the motion was lost [naturally].
The QATB had a responsibility with First aid instruction as the QATB A/O had to accept the patient from the First aider so it behove the QATB to have some input.

E. Bradley State secretary requested his speech from the Superintendent but as it was spontaneous, the Superintendent had to write up what he had spoken and submitted same to the State Council Secretary.

QATB GATTON.

1973 The six years at Gatton where there was a high road trauma rate allowed testing of staff education and training, and the time for setting the scene for future pre-hospital emergency care by qualified Ambulance officers – staff training :-

- at Centre by the Supt.
- at Hospital by Doctors
- In Theatre for airway management.

As a Founder Member of the IAO(Aust.) I used every advantage to further my philosophy, I used every opportunity to convince Medical personal, State Council and officers of the benefit to patients of ALS by A/o's and that Ambulance Officers were professionals.

Delegation.

As was my style I was totally involved in every aspect of Centre activities, (Superintendents were supposed to be 'on call' 24 hours a day).
I would attend to the administration during the day, but if there was an overload of cases and all staff out, I would attend that accident or transport leaving the Office assistant to answer the phone and relay calls.

If staff were busy I would assist them to clean and restock their Unit etc.

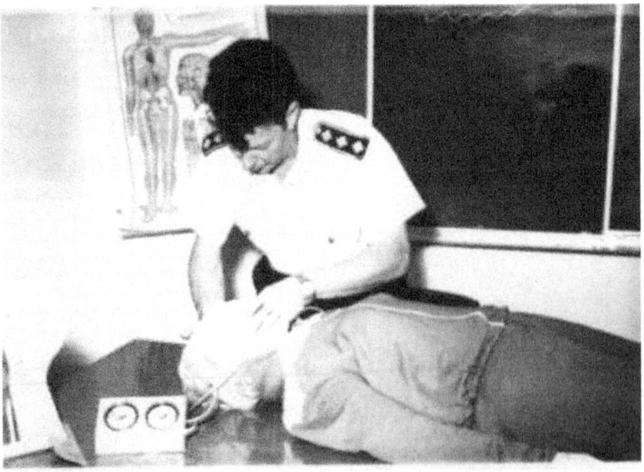

Regular First Aid courses were conducted at Gatton Centre.

After 6pm. I would attend as the first response to any emergency within 5 minutes of the Centre and the 'on-call' Officer would be called in to meet me 'at scene' to assist and continue with the case.

It was due to my assisting my officers that I made the decision to delegate.

I was washing a Unit whilst an officer was having his lunch before transporting a case to a Brisbane hospital when I twisted my back and suffered what is commonly called 'a slipped disc' which put me in hospital for some days.

This taught me that you cannot do everything, you must leave certain responsibilities to others. The way to ensure the tasks were satisfactorily completed was to train staff in their respective roles and to support this with clear written procedures.

Random, quiet, personal supervisory inspections maintain quality assurance and keep you aware of excellence or dereliction of duties - this is a must.

Delegation of duties is a compromise - it means that some tasks will not be completed to as high a standard as you would have done, and some may be carried out in a different but more efficient manner than you might have done.

This caused some Superintendents to 'hold onto' some admin tasks in case the junior staff member did a better job of it than the Super and impressed the committee - I believed that a good manager should always be looking for staff with 'promise' and should quietly direct them by developing their abilities -

good management is choosing the right person for the appropriate task and briefing them thoroughly on your requirements; if 'they' want to do it - give 'them' a go.

RESEARCH INTO BASIC EMERGENCY TREATMENT FOR SUB CRANIAL HAEMORRHAGE.

As an administrator, operational manager or Superintendent, it does not matter what organisation or business you are responsible for, you must conduct research into new methods for delivery of service to ensure the organisation maintains its high standard.

I virtually thought Ambulance practice and patient care 24 hours a day, so there was always some aspect of technique or treatment that was under examination by my subconscious mind, what we could do to control sub cranial haemorrhage in the time it took to reach definitive medical aid was one of these conundrums.
I read somewhere that the Japanese were using ice packs to control / reduce sub-cranial haemorrhage?? Would this work??

I called on the local butcher and told him I needed a shoulder blade with some meat left on the one surface of the flat blade and the underside clean for a project.
He didn't hesitate, he trimmed a beef shoulder blade to my specifications and wrapped it up, no charge - you see he was used to supplying me with the odd heart or long bone sawn down the centre to show the hard bone and matrix layers etc for lectures I gave to staff and the public.

I returned to the Centre and set up for my experiment. I taped a thermometer to the cleaner underside of the flat part of the blade, the sub cranial surface. Then placed a single layer of woollen material (pseudo hair) over the fleshy top side of the blade and bandaged an ice pack on top of this without obstructing the thermometer, and stood the whole on its side so that I could note the graduations.
Within a few minutes the thermometer showed a drop in temperature, the cold of the ice pack quickly penetrated the thickness of flesh and flat bone. Of course there was no circulation of warm blood to counteract the cold effect, but then again in the shocked situation the blood pressure drops anyway.

Now that I had demonstrated that an ice pack would significantly reduce the temperature of the sub cranial surface, I wrote to the Japanese Ambulance Service through the Consulate in Tokyo asking for any information on this procedure so that I would have some positive evidence to support introduction of a trial treatment - I received no reply.

I did speak to a couple of Doctors about this technique but received only negative responses so I too ceased following this line because [at that time] the Medical hierarchy of the Health Department did not treat kindly to any initiative other than from senior Medical officers.

THE FIRST AMBULANCE SEMINAR IN QUEENSLAND – December of 1975

The Institute of Ambulance Officers of Australia had been established for about 3 years when I attended the National meeting in Melbourne in 1975, but instead of attending the official Dinner on the Saturday night I had arranged to 'run' with the MICA, [Mobile Intensive Care Ambulance], emergency crew, so I spent the night 'on the road' and at the Hospital Emergency Department, but I learned a lot about this new service and their training curriculum; I met their Coronary Care Instructor, Carolyn Carlisle, who was a Queenslander, and was to be home in Toowoomba for Christmas.

Opportunity not only has to be recognised, but you must grasp it and run with it.

I asked her if she would be willing to give a presentation on the Victorian Coronary Care program to a seminar in Gatton whilst she was on holidays, she gave an enthusiastic 'yes'- *now all I had to do was to go home and organise it !!!*

Planning commenced from that moment so that the day after my return to Gatton I was on the move, I spoke to my good friend Bob Spearritt the Principal of the Gatton High School, who gave permission for me to use the Assembly Hall for the Seminar during the School holidays.
Val said the Ambulance Ladies Committee would cater for the Lunch and morning tea for the Seminar.

I knew that the Gatton Committee would support any action for improving the knowledge of officers so the chat with Alan Muller, my Chairman, was really only one of communication.

I intended to run the Seminar as an Institute activity but when I rang and spoke with Reg Bartels the Superintendent of Brisbane Centre and the Chairman of the Queensland Division I met with opposition to the project, Reg not only was not in favour he was against any Institute involvement - such was the negative thinking on progressive procedures for Ambulance by most of the senior Superintendents.

I then informed him and Jack McMasters, Super of Ipswich, that I intended to conduct this Seminar no matter what, and I was simply giving the Institute the opportunity to take the credit - finally Reg and Jack gave the OK for me to say the Seminar was under the auspices of the Institute, but the proviso was that 'Skippy' Davidson, Deputy Superintendent of Brisbane, be given an opportunity to speak.
We were away - I contacted Dr. Ian MacDonald from Toowoomba Hospital who had assisted the Ambulance at many a road accident on the Warrego Highway if he would speak on emergency procedures at the Road-side and on the need for Fluid replacement, he was only too happy to speak on one of his favourite topics, so the day was covered.

I rang Carolyn Carlisle to confirm dates re her holidays and availability for our Seminar, then drafted a Registration form, roneoed off about 200 copies, [we did not have a photocopier then, in fact no one did], and sent these out to Institute members throughout the State for them to copy and distribute.

On the 28th December 1975 the first State Seminar on Patient care and Emergency Procedures was conducted in Queensland with an attendance of 77 officers from throughout Queensland - a major step forward in the future of Pre-hospital emergency Patient Care by the Ambulance service.

TRANSCRIPTION of the OPENING ADDRESS of the first Institute Seminar in Qld. 28/12/1975, by the Chairman, Founder Member Malcolm McDonald.

Distinguished Guests, Members, Ladies and gentlemen.

It is with great pleasure that I give the opening address to this Seminar for the Institute of Ambulance Officers Queensland Division, doubly so in that this is the first Seminar to be held by the Institute in Queensland.

It is most gratifying to see such a large attendance here today, when one considers the adverse conditions, and the time of year.
The adverse conditions of widespread wet weather which has preceded this day, causing travelling to be most inconvenient and troublesome, the festive season where you have conflicting loyalties to your family and home, and the period of time when the workload of most Centres is at its peak; so that the attendance here today reflects on the deep interest you have in the Institute, the dedication to your service, and your hopes in its future progress.

The inception of the Institute of Ambulance Officers Australia would be one of the greatest steps forward in the history of the Ambulance Service in Australia since that Service had its humble beginning at the Queensland Exhibition in the late 1800's, when a few men saw the need and the necessity for some organisation to be available to help relieve the suffering of their fellow man.
Further meetings were held so that the first Ambulance Service in Australia was inaugurated, and took its Training from the manual of the Queensland Defence Forces Ambulance Corps. Certainly the Ambulance Service is "A Broadening Field" when you look at the rich harvest which has resulted from the early nurture and care rendered by those first dedicated men.

The aims of the Institute is to forever uphold the ethics of the profession, to always strive for a greater knowledge and understanding, and to work with dedication to even further improve on every facet of the service as we know it today.
It is also the duty of the Institute to be an open Forum for discussion of all matters brought forward by medical research or medical practitioners, anything which is

relevant to the Ambulance Service, even if this may be of a slightly controversial nature, for it is only with free and open discussion of the various aspects put forward by different men that we can hope to move forward and not stagnate.

These ideas may be at times either radical or only mediocre, but with discussion, the radical ideas can be tempered down and the mediocre uplifted to techniques which could and would be of great assistance and benefit to the people we serve.

For we must never lose sight of the actual reason for the Ambulance Service, that of "patient care." Patient Care must always, and is always at the forefront of our thinking, everything we do must be towards this end, so that if techniques are available to relieve suffering and to sustain life, then, if we do not use them, we are only a second class service and must be conscious of this fact.

It is the duty of each one of us as Institute members to sacrifice our time, to bring forward our hopes and ideas, to be positive in our thinking, always looking to better ways of serving the sick and injured, yet never changing simply for the sake of change alone. NB: original paper available.

Malcolm C McDonald

Doctor Ian MacDonald presented a most informative and educational paper on "The Value of Infusion in the Pre-Hospital situation," relating to patients with Shock from trauma and on their need for fluid replacement etc.

Carolyn Carlisle then gave a presentation on the different fluids available for infusion, their composition, what conditions they were most suited for, and contraindications for fluid replacement; after lunch she presented papers on the MICA service in Victoria and on Coronary Care training.

The officers were left with a new appreciation of what was available 'out there' and what could be done for 'the patient.'
Deputy Superintendent Davidson was given the opportunity to thank the Speakers and to say a few words, he moved an appropriate vote of thanks but then concluded by saying, "but let us not forget that the First Aid Book is our guide and prompt first aid is the most important aspect of Ambulance work"- you could almost hear the chaps saying, 'yeah! yeah!'

I had organised staff to record the full presentations on tape and now came the huge task of transcribing this, Val typed from the tape with my assistance, then we copied the pages on the Roneo machine and sent a full copy to all who attended so that the message was reinforced and passed on to other officers, ***the move forward for improved pre-hospital care had gained impetus.***

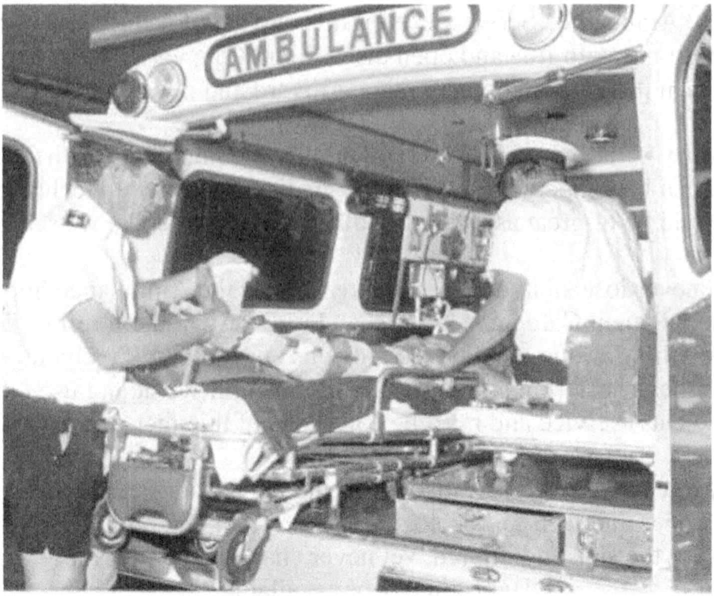

Supt. McDonald applies a Thomas splint to a 'patient' with SAO Harding assisting.

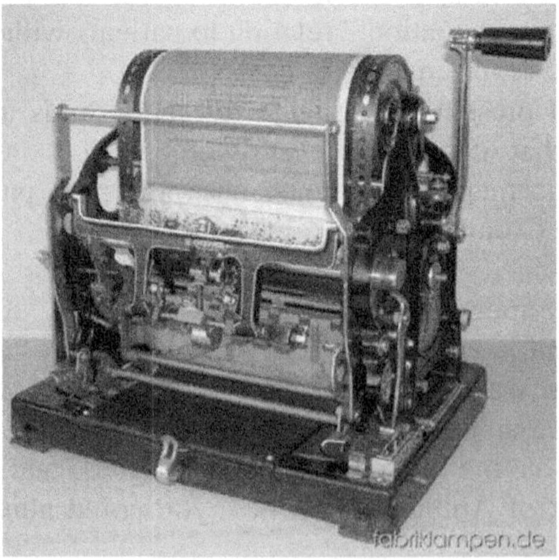

Roneo copying machine.

THE BIG DROP.

After the day's work I had not long gone to bed when the phone woke me at 11 pm. The caller said, "a car or truck has crashed through the Tent Hill creek bridge and down into the creek".

"How many injured?" I asked "I dun know mate, but it's a bloody long way to the creek-bed!" he replied.
"Righto we'll be on our way," I said.

Val had woken also, "what's the problem?" I was changing into white overalls, "ring Pat, he's on-call, tell him to come in and to stand by, I'm going to Tent Hill bridge to check out a report that a car has crashed off it into the creek."

I left in a F100 emergency unit, and arrived at the bridge in five minutes, stopped on the bridge with red beacon and four flashing side lights operating, engine still running, and looked over the broken side rail of the bridge.

At least 40 foot below lay a wrecked truck, upright, in about a foot of water in the creek bed. Two people were near the front cabin, so I asked if anyone was in the vehicle? and if so how were they?

A faint call back, "one bloke seems to hurt bad, and eh can't get out, he's trapped".

"Tell him the Ambulance is here and I'll be down in a minute".

I drove to the end of the bridge and parked off the road, I radioed the centre, my on-call ambulance officer had arrived and answered, I informed him of the situation, then instructed him to collect our Major Emergency box which contained nylon ropes, reflective vests, some rescue gear, heavy duty torches and supply of dressings and bandages, and to bring extra ropes for lowering gear.
Further instruction was in accordance with our set procedures for an entrapment, that he was to set up support on the bridge, protected by all warning lights and Police on scene.

I asked Val to stand by at the radio in case we required further assistance.

I climbed, (slipped and stumbled) down the creek bank, ambulance kit in one hand, torch and gear in the other, in the dark, as the torch was not much help after the first slip.
The truck was extensively damaged as it had struck the bank first and then rolled into the creek bed to come to rest on twisted wheels facing the bridge, driver's side against the water eroded creek bank.

The doors were buckled, the hood dented, the front and bonnet dented and bent. I was able to stand on the flat creek bank and look through the driver's window.

I found the driver conscious but trapped by the bent steering column forcing the steering wheel against his right thigh – I reassured him.

"You'll be right, we'll check things out and then get you out and to a Doctor – now, where does it hurt?"
I assessed the driver and found that he had some small lacerations to the face and arms, pain to the cervical and lumbar spine which I classed as possible fractures, a fracture to the thigh under the steering wheel.

He was conscious with regular breathing, presenting with the early signs of shock.

On finding the probable cervical spine, I immediately applied a cervical collar to his neck - "that's to protect your neck and to ease the pain".

I sent a bystander up to my unit for the Entonox for pain relief.

I informed my patient that further assistance was on its way.

Extrication was going to be difficult due to the damage to the vehicle and because it was hard against the eroded bank.

A/O Pat Denham my back-up had arrived and there were about six willing helpers down in the creek bed by this, one being a Police officer.
I instructed Pat to lower the Emergency box over the bridge rail, using the extra ropes he had brought as part of the equipment.

The Entonox come down first so I instructed my patient on its use for pain relief and how to use it, on his second inhalation I carried on.

I informed the Police officer of the patient's condition, and discussed the best method to extricate the patient.

I said, "I've got to be able to reach him and lift him out somehow, so we can start by cutting the cabin supports, then pulling the cabin roof back".

The Emergency box had been lowered, and as we removed the ropes, torches and the most needed metal saw with its spare blades.

Sketch of the night patient rescue carried out at Tent Hill Ck.

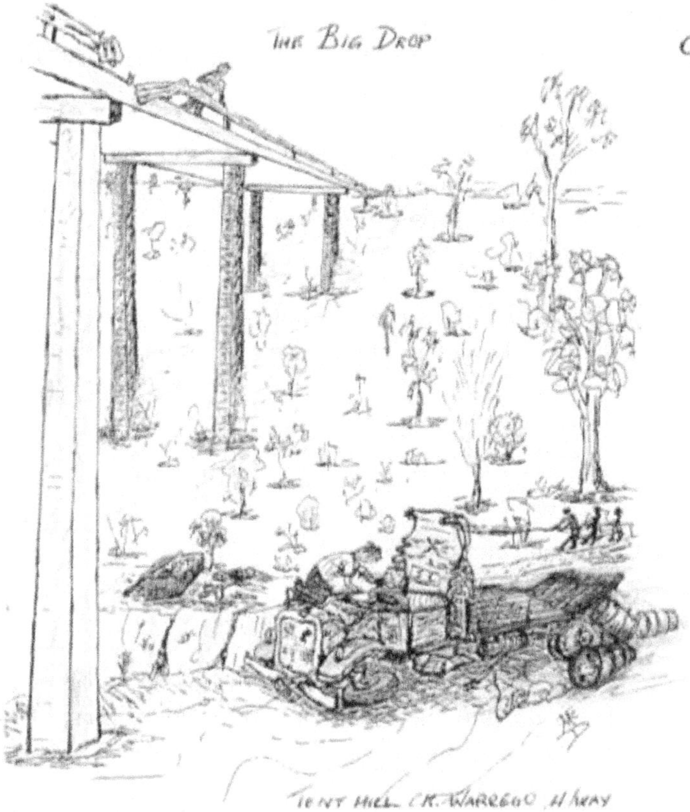

Initial contact and primary assessment of the patient.

Out of the darkness of the steep bank came a call, “do you need a hand?” followed by the figure of Dr. Ian MacDonald from Toowoomba.
Ian was a supporter of the Ambulance, and had presented a paper on The Value of Infusion in the Pre-Hospital situation, at a Seminar I had organised at Gatton in December of 1975.

Dr MacDonald was a practical person and would always stop to assist at accidents even if it was to use tools to assist in extrication - I introduced Dr. MacDonald to the patient.

I left the Police officer to organise the rescue party, and to implement any request for equipment or specific action, while Ian and myself attended to the patient and the problem of his safe removal.
Using the metal hand saw, helpers cut through the windscreen supports and cabin struts, the Police officer then organised ropes tied to these, and with a number of men on each rope pulling back over the cabin, they pulled the cabin roof backwards folding it along a indent from the smash, allowing easy access to our patient from above.

I informed the patient that we were going to remove the steering wheel, and instructed him to breathe up on the Entonox for pain relief, "we'll have you out shortly", I told him.

Ian and I then cut through the steering wheel spokes, close to the column, thereby removing the wheel without danger of the rim springing, thus releasing the pressure on our patient's fractured thigh and allowing us to move to the next phase of his actual removal from the smashed vehicle.

Our problem was that we had a patient with probable spinal injuries, a definite fractured right thigh, sitting in the vehicle, below our working level and we had to remove him without causing any further injury ???.

We decided that the only way was by lifting him straight up, but how? In this restricted space and uneven terrain.

I had the answer, I discussed it with Ian who gave it the nod.

My support officer had climbed down the steep bank and joined us.
I informed him what I required and what had to be done.

I told our patient what we intended to do, and that I wanted him to stay calm and not to try to help by pushing or holding on to anything.

Pat handed me a blanket rolled lengthways, this I threaded under the patients right arm from behind, across his chest, then under his left arm, then carefully adjusted the length until I had to two ends of the blanket up behind the patient's neck.

Pat handed Ian the end of a rope and Ian tied the ends of the blanket together at the level of his shoulders, (Ian's hobby was sailing).

I told the Police officer what I needed and he called two strong helpers over, one climbed up onto the bonnet with him and the other stood on the top of the seat behind the patient.

Pat had prepared the light rescue stretcher and stood on the bank beside the cabin with two helpers each side, holding the stretcher.

On my instruction, "take the strain, now lift", the Police officer and the two helpers pulled the rope up vertically, Ian and myself did our best to support the injured thigh as the patient was lifted bodily upwards.

As he came free of the wrecked cabin other willing hands helped with the awkward lift, with a command of -

"CAREFUL! KEEP HIM STRAIGHT AND ONLY LIFT ON THE BLANKET!"

"It's going fine mate," I said to the patient.

As soon as his feet were clear, "right Pat closer with the stretcher."
Pat and his helpers held the stretcher upright, "now chaps turn him - closer Pat – that's it, against the stretcher, now hold him - lower it like a hinge."
As the patient was lowered to the narrow strip of bank there was a spontaneous shout from the group for a job well done.

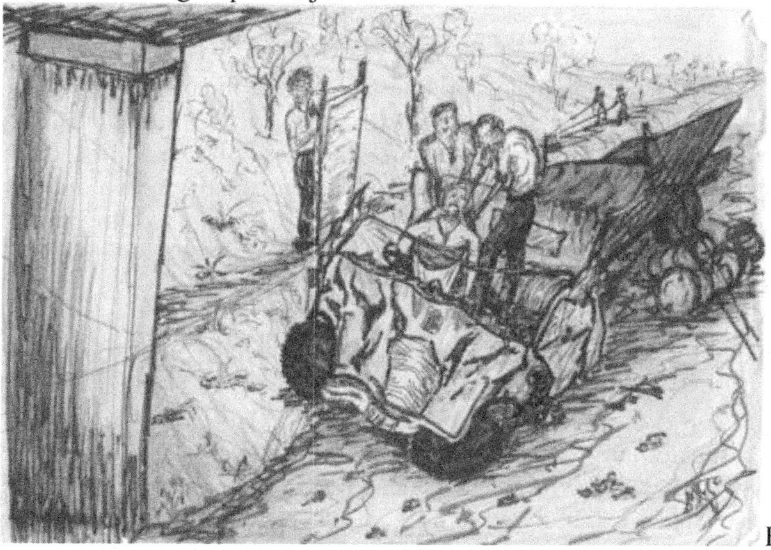

EXTRICATION
Sketch of the smashed truck in Tent Hill creek bed.

BUT we weren't finished yet.

Pat applied a Thomas splint to the fractured thigh, I assisted and Dr. Ian MacDonald reassessed the patient's condition.

The next job was to get our patient up the steep bank.
I asked the Police officer to organise a party for this job.

Pat tied ropes to each of the four corners of the stretcher, then a long rope to the top. The patient was then tied to the stretcher with sheets, one across his chest another across his knees and legs.

The Police officer organised a two men to climb the bank with the long rope and to keep tension on it at all times. Two men each side lifting the stretcher, others holding ropes tied to the rear corners - and up we started.

Even with all these helpers the stretcher tilted and rocked as one then another

slipped or lost their grip, but others took up the slack and we reached the top and road level at last, it had been an exhausting climb and carry.
I looked at my watch, 1am in the morning!
I haven't told Val how things were, **she'll still be at the radio!**

I hurried over to the car, called Gatton Centre, Val answered straight away in a very tired voice, "VL 4IV Gatton control"
I informed her of the situation and said we'd be loading and then to transporting to Gatton Hospital so, "all's well, you can go back to bed now", I received a very brief, "thanks".

We loaded our patient and Dr. MacDonald said he would infuse the patient.
I selected the bottle of S.P.P.S. and the giving set, I grasped the 'bull' needle to puncture the rubber stopper in the bottle, oops remove the foil cover first, then connected the apparatus, checked the flow to fill the tubing and remove any air bubbles, and handed the end tube to Dr. McDonald who had cannulated the patient and was ready to connect the infusion set to him.
Tape it in place, short arm splint, off to Gatton hospital.

Another case completed, with the satisfaction of a 'job well done' and something achieved.

The patient was later transferred to Toowoomba hospital then to Princess Alexandra Hospital the next day. He had suffered 2 cervical fractures, 1 dorsal fracture, 1 lumber fracture, and a fractured right femur.

He sustained a fat embolism on the fifth day, but he was finally discharged with no major physical defects.

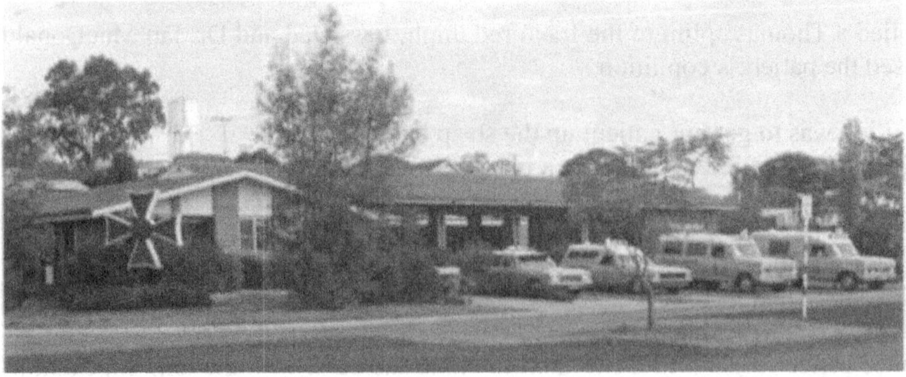

QATB Gatton Centre 1974 – note F100 Units on the style introduced by Supt. Doug Henning of Toowoomba. My innovation was for the cupboard for dressings and appliances had to be clear Perspex so that all was visible as a reminder of what was available for use.

Monitor/ defibrillator NO! NO! NEVER! – the state of play in 1976.

By late 1975 Gatton was one of the most up to date Centres in Queensland with well trained staff through the Q.A.T.B. Training School and from regular lectures conducted at the hospital, as well as a structured skills maintenance program.
The Ford F100 Ambulance Units carried resuscitation equipment of Oxy Viva and Air Viva, Aspiration units, oxygen therapy gear, transfusion kits, S.P.P.S. and Haemacell fluids and Entonox.
As well as the "Doctor's use only Kit" containing: - laryngoscope, various endotracheal tubes, Spencer-Wells forceps, 'liquorice stick connector,' syringes and cannula etc.

The local hospital had a Medical Superintendent with the right to private practise who attended at the hospital for morning outpatients, specific procedures and was called as required for emergencies.

The Ambulance centre attended many calls of 'chest pain' from muscular, pulmonary, skeletal, peptic or cardiac origin.
Most calls were after six in the evening from a patient suffering 'chest pain.' Sometimes the origin was obvious with the pain pattern identifiable and definite but in the majority of cases there was always some doubt.

As Gatton serviced mainly a country district on an average it could take the Ambulance 30 minutes from time of call to reach the patient, another 15 minutes plus to access, ready, stretcher and load the patient into the unit, then a further 30 minutes to the hospital.
The Doctor would take 10 minutes to arrive – the charge Sister had to check the patient first – another 20 minutes for the examination and assessment of the patient and a letter for the Specialist at Toowoomba – 45 to 60 minutes to travel to Toowoomba hospital.

In all of this time there was NO PROGRESSIVE CARDIAC RECORD of the patient's condition – A CARDIAC ARREST COULD BE IMMINENT but there was nothing to warn of this except the sudden collapse of the patient which was a bit late to say the least.

My opinion was that if the patient had a simple ECG trace recorded with name date and time when the ambulance arrived, and 30 minutes later on arrival at Gatton hospital another activation of the monitor for a second tracing. The local Doctor could note if there was no cardiac history, or, that the patient should be transferred to Toowoomba when a third tracing could be recorded 45 to 60 minutes later on arrival.
If this procedure was introduced the receiving Specialist would have a PROGRESSIVE CARDIAC RECORD of, 30, 60 and 135/150 minutes from the time the ambulance attended the case of 'chest pain' thus providing valuable

information for the Specialist to make an informed diagnosis and if required to immediately initiate lifesaving treatment.

In July 1976, with the approval of the Gatton Ambulance Committee I called a meeting of the local Doctors with the Committee to discuss and decide on procedures to provide Pre-hospital cardiac Care to the people of the Gatton district from: Ambulance to Doctor to Specialist to hospital.
The proposal was for Gatton Ambulance Officers be trained to prepare and attach the three electrode leads to the patient, to activate the monitor and to run an ECG trace. Safety procedures and basic machine mechanics were also required knowledge.
Any further use of the machine was under the Doctor's control, Ambulance Officers were not to proceed past taking an ECG reading.

The three local Doctors agreed with and supported this proposal and offered to train officers in the necessary procedure with a Certificate of competence on completion of the course.

I then organised a demonstration of the monitoring machine for the Gatton Rotary Club which supported my proposal by promising $4000 dollars to purchase such a machine.

In October the Honourable Dr. Lew Edwards, the Minister for Health visited Gatton centre and was impressed with standard of Pre-hospital patient care administered by officers and the progressive emergency procedures in place as well as those under development.

In the annual budget I included the purchase of a Monitor/ defibrillator from the QATB Gatton Trust Fund to use money donated by the Rotary Club for that specific purpose.
The rationale for this was provided in detail.

I was more than surprised to receive a reply through the Medical Adviser to the Q.A.T.B. State Council that this was not approved but also vetoing the purchase and use of such a Machine.
This was most definite, to the extent of officially stating :-
"No Queensland Ambulance car shall carry this equipment ~~."

I was so astounded by this totally negative and stagnant attitude from the Medical Adviser that I replied to the Secretary of the Q.A.T.B. State Council:- " I have received the reply to my proposal for the Gatton Q.A.T.B. to purchase a Monitor/ defibrillator that: "no ambulance shall carry such equipment," and I find this statement so negative that I can only conclude it was a typographical error.

I despatched this in the full knowledge that my promotional chances would be jeopardised for the next three or so years but I believed an official protest had to be lodged.

The introduction of Advanced Life Support procedures for use by Q.A.T.B. officers was prevented by the ultra conservatism of certain senior State Medical personnel in areas of influence at that time.
It was to take to July of 1986 for the Q.A.T.B. to finally introduce Pre-hospital Coronary Care.

It was a long time from 1976 to 1986.

I took up my appointment as Superintendent Q.A.T.B. Ipswich in November of 1979 with a 5 year plan to lift the Pre-hospital patient care from basic first-aid to the provision of Advanced Life Support.

This is outlined in a later chapter.

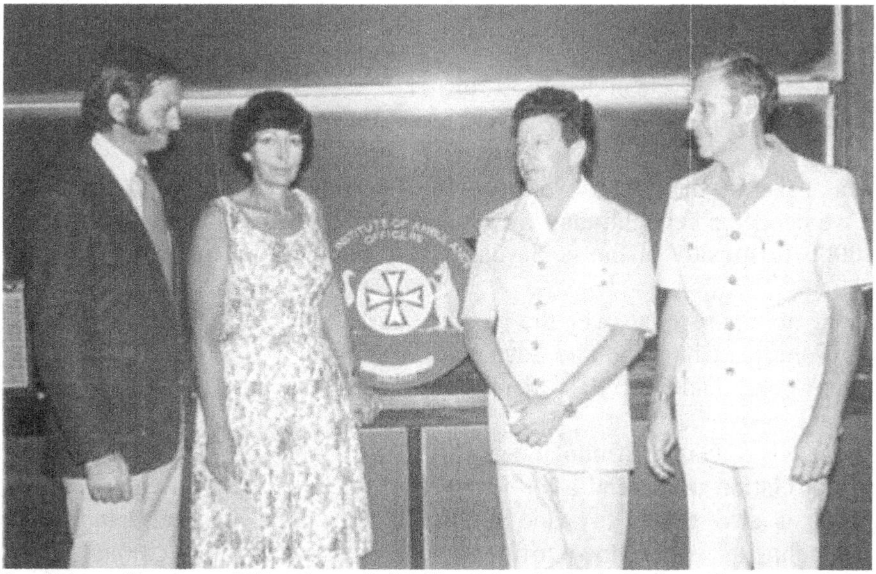

Seminar Gatton: DR. Darryl Wall, PA. Spinal Unit; Charge RN. Boyd, PA Hospital; Supt. McDonald; Dr. Noel Stevenson, Director Casualty Dept. Princess Alexandra Hospital.

RESCUE and TRANSPORT. FOUR BY FOUR CAN EQUAL ONE.

Lochy Rule, a member of the Lion's Cabinet, came to me one day in 1979 and offered $10,000 to the Ambulance for a new vehicle, he said that it had become available for Gatton because the Ipswich Superintendent had been offered the donation but Jack McMaster had said Ipswich did not need one - *but there was a proviso.*

The Lion's cabinet, the State body, had identified a need for Ambulance to have Rescue Units with equipment to extricate victims from crashed vehicles involved in road smashes or whatever.
To assist they had initiated a project where they would donate $10000 to appropriate Centres to be used for the provision of a Rescue Unit.

I had heard of this project because Doug Henning, Super of Toowoomba Centre had already accepted the Lion's donation and were building a fully equipped Rescue Unit on a Range Rover chassis.

I immediately said, "Yes Lochy, the Gatton Committee will accept the Lion's donation for a Rescue Unit, but come back to me in three days and I will have some ideas on such a Unit, and we can discuss it further,"
again, ***one takes the opportunity when it is offered.***

I had no idea at that moment as to what sought of a Unit we might build, but I was certain that we needed a new Unit and we needed the money, [$10000 donation gave another $10000 in subsidy in the next year], so it was now up to me to put it all together.
I gave it all of my spare time over the next couple of days, had a chat with Alan Muller the Committee Chairman and got his blessing, so that when Lochy called on me later in the week, I had my project ready for him.

I outlined the needs of Gatton Ambulance.
I explained that Gatton did attend a lot of road accidents on the Warrego Highway especially, but it also served a wide district where farm workers had tractor accidents, parachutists were blown off course and fell into hilly country, bush walkers were injured in inaccessible country, so that Gatton required a Rescue Unit which could attend to different types of rescue in differing terrain, the ideal being a 4 wheel drive vehicle.

Secondly Gatton did not have high staff numbers, and if we needed a 4 wheel drive Rescue Unit to get to a patient, then that Unit had to be capable of transporting the patient also, it had to be a Rescue /treat and transport Unit.

This could be manufactured as an F100 Ford Ambulance, [with 4 wheel drive], with storage and access to specific rescue equipment, and with some medical equipment and one stretcher for a patient.

Lochy agreed with my proposal, asked me to put it in writing, and he would attend to the presentation of the cheque - shortly after the Gatton Committee received the $10000 donation for a new Rescue Unit.

It did not take long for me to plan a suitable and versatile Unit, I had planned renovations for the first F100 Units previously purchased so I simply rearranged and substituted.

The Rescue /treat and Transport Unit would have side cupboards for medical gear which were accessible from the outside and inside; a full height cupboard was made to house crow bar, shovel, axe, ropes, sledge hammer and cutting chisels etc.

Other side cupboards held hydraulic 'spreaders' and the 'jaws of life,' as well as lighting equipment; the front bumper bar was a water tank and had an electric winch attached. The spare stretcher base was constructed with cross bars so it could be used as a ladder, etc.
The only disagreement I had with the Committee in our discussions on my proposals was with the actual 4 wheel drive. The Chairman suggested it be automatic - I did not agree on the grounds that as a Rescue Unit reliability was of the essence and power in low gear would be a factor in a number of rescues.
I was overruled and the resolution was for an automatic F100 4x4 Ford chassis be ordered for the base of the Rescue Unit.

The next day I rang Southside Ford in Brisbane and asked if they had a chassis available and if I could come in to check same - affirmative on both counts.
I took our mechanic with me and went in to check the automatic out; when I arrived at Southside Ford I noticed the high embankment of the Freeway behind their workshop.

I explained what we wanted and what the vehicle would be used for; Ross Harding our mechanic asked very searching questions as to power, gear ratios etc, until we were satisfied theoretically.
I then looked outside at the steep embankment and asked if I could test the vehicle on the slope ? "go right ahead," the salesman replied.

I drove the 4x4 outside and around to the embankment and carefully faced it up the steep slope and stopped.
I put it into drive and gently accelerated, it took it like a baby drinks milk, I felt more apprehensive of the steep angle than the vehicle, but I had tested it to my satisfaction, and I was now happy to accept that it could do the job I wanted it to do - *if it's going to be your responsibility, then check the facts thoroughly.*

We ordered the Ford F100 4x4 automatic model.

Ron Dallas of Superior Body Works accepted our plans and gave an acceptable quote. The Rescue Unit was built and put into service to attend all road accidents as a first response Unit.
It was most successful in its role and a major asset in Rescue providing reduced timeframe for getting our patients to definitive Medical care.

It was the first 4x4 Ambulance in Queensland capable of Rescue/ Treat and Transport.

THE 4X4 ATTENDS ITS FIRST ACCIDENT:

The day the new Unit was put into service it was used to attend a 2 car road accident near the QAC on the Warrego Highway; on arrival I found the driver of one car with a severe laceration to her forehead and trapped in the vehicle. The driver of the other vehicle was found wandering around in a dazed condition suffering concussion and possible internal injuries.

One officer guided the one driver to the Ambulance unit, whilst I attended the trapped victim and directed the extrication of the trapped patient, Dr. Ian MacDonald walked over to me, [he frequently travelled the Warrego Highway from Toowoomba to Brisbane and back], he offered his assistance.
As the only injury the Doctor could access was the laceration, he gave his attention to the extrication of the trapped patient.

As I administered emergency treatment I learned that the patient's father was a member of Lions in Brisbane, so coincidentally the first patient to benefit from the Rescue Unit was the daughter of a Lion Club member.

Yes the four by four Rescue Unit did equal one "well cared for patient."

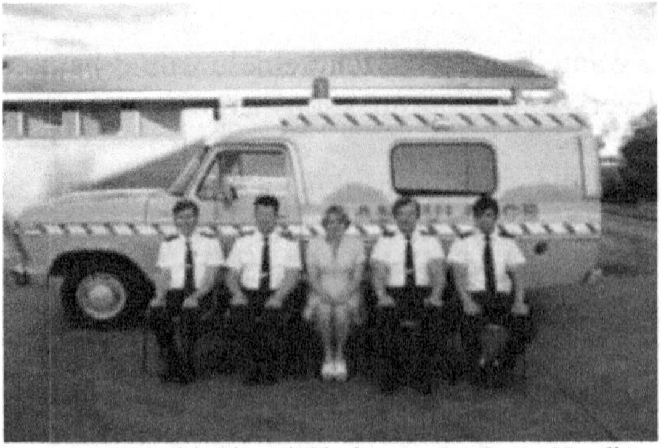

AO. P. Denham, Supt. McDonald; Sheryl Chalmers; SAO. R. Harding; AO. R. Fletcher.

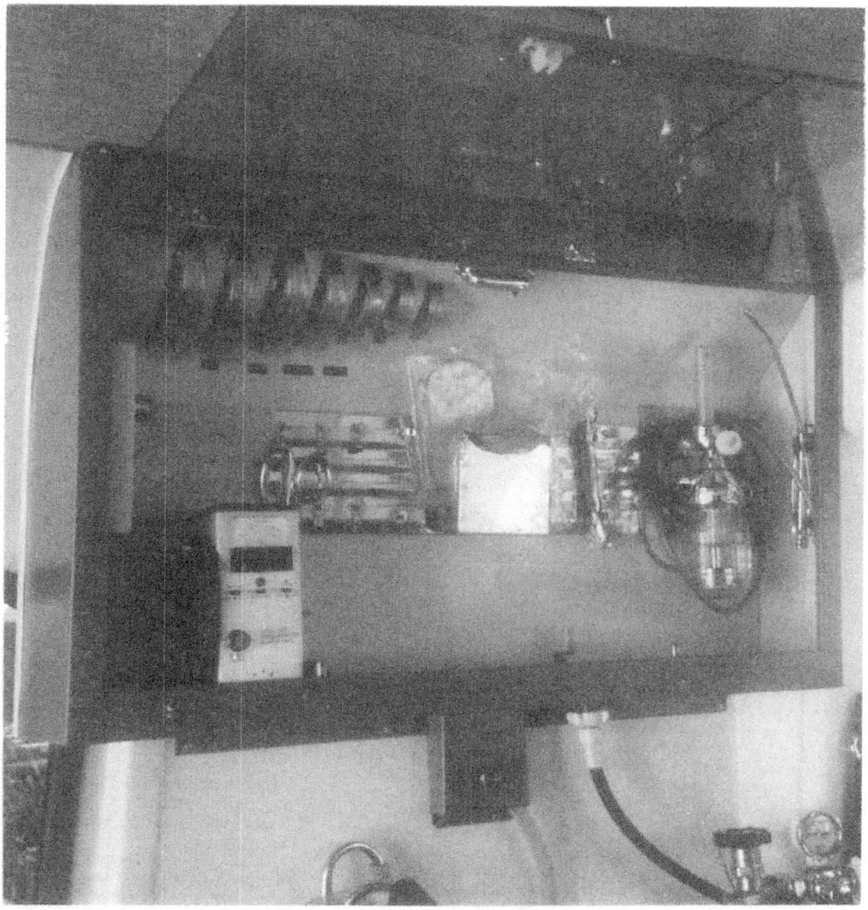

1979 Resuscitation equipment in Unit

QUEENSLAND TIMES. 10/9/79.

Go-anywere unit for Gatton QATB

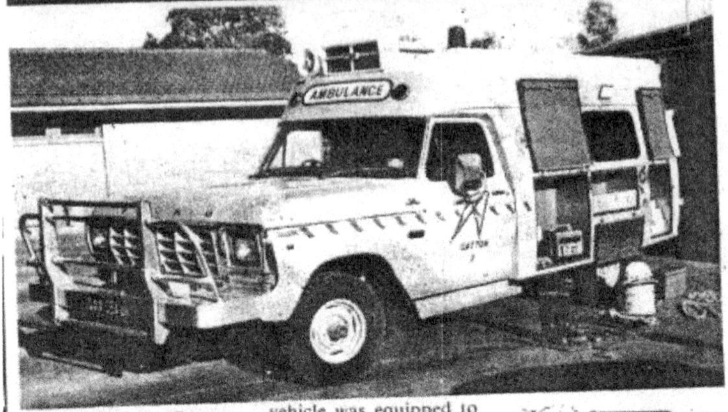

GATTON — **Gatton Ambulance Centre now has in operation a unit — the first of its kind in Queensland — considered to be the best equipped available.**

The unit, pictured below, was handed over to the Gatton Centre by Gatton Lions' Club president, Mr G. Simpson at the club's annual ball on Friday night. 7/9/79.

Cost $25,000

The ambulance has been purchased at a cost of $25,000 and of this Gatton Lions donated $10,000. The Ambulance Centre raised $5000 and subsidy was $10,000.

Receiving the car keys, Mr Mal McDonald, the Gatton Centre superintendent, said it was certainly Gatton Lions Club's greatest effort as far as Gatton Ambulance was concerned. The ambulance had been very fortunate in that the three service clubs in Gatton had all played their part in helping to maintain the service.

He said the new vehicle was equipped to meet any emergency likely to be encountered in the district, and having four-wheel drive, it could travel to areas at present inaccessible to standard vehicles.

The main function of the vehicle would be rescue, treat, and transport, with further treatment during transport.

Mr McDonald said an ambulance in the Gatton area required the capacity to treat cases on a main highway, with heavy inbound and outbound traffic 20 hours a day. Mountainous areas surrounding the town; inaccessible areas where trail bike riders and bush walkers had been injured in the past; light wooded paddocks, where rescue of a parachutist or horse riding accidents could need ambulance help.

Equipment

Mr McDonald said the vehicle submitted to and chosen by the Lions was capable of meeting all these needs.

For the case of a patient being at the base of a hill or over a cliff, a rescue stretcher with ropes and pulleys was carried.

An Eni-a-pack hydraulic lifting and spreading tool was in the equipment, with saw chisels etc for cutting, as well as bars, shovels and picks to reach debris victims.

All officers of Gatton Ambulance have attended the QATB State Council school stages 1 and 2, and Superintendent McDonald recently attended the specialised stage 3.

COUNTRY SECTION

THE PROFESSIONAL KICK OFF – from BLS to ALS.

Progression of appointments provided the opportunity to gain knowledge and experience as the base to introduce improvements in patient care.

My appointment as Superintendent to Wowan centre in 1969 was the culmination of 14 years experience. From 4 years as First Aid attendant in the Qld. Railway, 3 years Honorary at Q.A.T.B. Cairns and with the Aerial Ambulance, then 7 years service as a Permanent officer placed me in a position with no local Doctor and (to me) the responsibility to meet the need to provide adequate Pre-hospital care to the people within the Q.A.T.B. Wowan District.

This gave me invaluable experience in working closely under the instruction of the Medical Superintendent of Mt. Morgan Hospital in advancing the Ambulance Casualty Room treatments, to dispensing drugs and administering various injections under his authority and controlled by his inspection every fortnight when he conducted a 'Doctors Clinic' at the Centre.
As a young Superintendent I applied for a place on the first Course of the new Q.A.T.B. Training School – this cemented my knowledge and skills.

The 1972 appointment to Maleny Ambulance District placed me closer to the decision making and availability to attend State meetings – it also gave me space to gain experience in diplomacy and managing resources.
The Centre Inspection by Commissioner Self and State Council members was an unexpected and successful examination of my Administration expertise and efficiency of delivering a reputable Ambulance Service.

The Inaugural meeting of the Institute of Ambulance Officers (Aust.) in Canberra 1973 was a major step towards professionalism – McDonald a Founder Member

1973: The six years at Gatton where there was a high road trauma rate was the opportunity to test the program for staff education and training, and the time for setting the criteria for the training of future Pre-hospital Emergency Care by qualified Ambulance officers:-

- At Centre by the Superintendent.
- At Hospital by Doctors
- In Theatre for airway management.

The Gatton Doctors, Rosenberg, Hudson and Hendry, were all supportive of, and co-operated in Ambulance officer Training as outlined by Supt. McDonald.

As a Founder Member of the of the IAO(Aust.) I used every advantage to further my philosophy that every patient had the right to receive best practise of Pre-hospital Emergency Care. I used every opportunity to convince Medical personal, State Council and Officers of the benefit to patients of ALS administered by Ambulance Officers. ref: Drs Hendry & Paul Rosenberg.

QUEENSLAND HOSPITALS

All Communications to be addressed to The Secretary.

In reply please quote this Number:

TOOWOOMBA *Hospitals Board.*

GATTON HOSPITAL
William Street,
GATTON 4343.

21st. September, 1979

The Secretary,
Q.A.T.B. State Council,
P.O. Box 272,
BROADWAY 4000.

Dear Sir,

I have been asked by MR. MALCOLM MC DONALD, Superintendent of the Gatton Q.A.T.B. to provide a reference for him which I am forwarding directly to you.

I have known Mr. McDonald since I took up my position as Medical Superintendent of Gatton Hospital approximately 10 months ago. During this time I have worked both with Mr. McDonald and members of his staff on many occasion. I have found the Gatton Q.A.T.B. to run efficiently, and I believe most of the credit for this must belong to Mr. McDonald himself. He is a very determined worker himself, but I think his greatest value is in his organizational ability and the way he is able to keep the Ambulance service here running at peak efficiency.

He is continually trying to education his officers and has allowed them to attend lectures given by myself at the hospital, and also to attend operating procedures so that they may learn more about resuscitation of the unconscious patient.

I have found his medical ethics to be beyond question, and at any time if I had any criticism of his service I have directed this to him and he has done his utmost to rectify the situation or improve my understanding of it.

I would be pleased to have someone with the qualities of Mr McDonald on my staff at any time.

Yours faithfully,

PAUL HENDRY
Medical Superintendent.

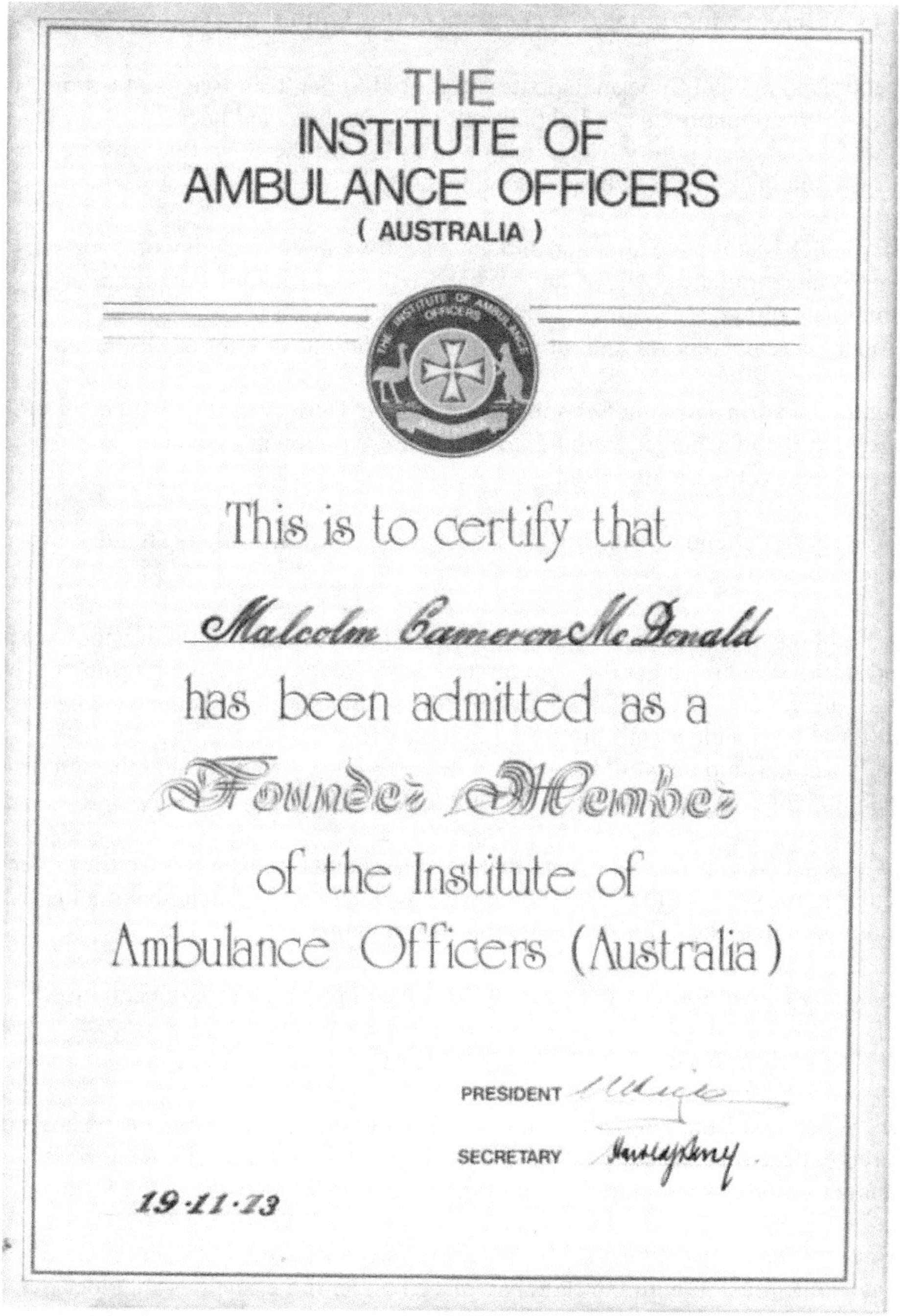

THE
INSTITUTE OF
AMBULANCE OFFICERS
(AUSTRALIA)

This is to certify that

Malcolm Cameron McDonald

has been admitted as a

Founder Member

of the Institute of
Ambulance Officers (Australia)

PRESIDENT

SECRETARY

19·11·73

1974 Conference in Victoria: "The Role of the Ambulance Officer."

I encouraged present Superintendents and retired Super Tom Briggs of Cairns fame to attend if I could organise a light aircraft to fly us there and back.
Lionel Blackman, a family friend, who was a pilot for the Bush Pilots offered to fly us down and back in a Cessna at a nominal cost.

THE WORKSHOP: We attended and gave positive input to each workshop on:- 'What is an ambulance officer' and 'What are the qualifications required' and 'What training is required.'
Coronary care procedures and intravenous cannulation were topics discussed.

I met the Victoria Training School Coronary Care Tutor [Caroline who came from Queensland] and arranged with her to give a presentation at a Seminar in Queensland , yet to be organised.

That evening I attended with MICA officers on cases while others attended the Conference Dinner.

The flight down was enjoyable and uneventful but the return flight did not have a good start. We arrived at the light aircraft aerodrome early in the morning to see a fogged-in airfield. There were some low hills within the flight path so we had to wait for at least a clear sighting for a safe take off.
Finally, Lionel said he would try a take off by flying a circuit around the aerodrome to gain height until he found an opening to exit.

This was sound in principle except that on our second circuit when we flew over a circular horse yard for the second time we saw a very irate owner shaking his fist at us and mouthing abuse for disturbing his thoroughbreds.

Thankfully Lionel found a faint gap in the fog and powered through and up.

THE INFLUENCE OF EMERGENCY TREATMENTS IN VIETNAM:

The "Scoop and Run" procedure advocated by some Trauma Surgeons wherein the injured patient was basically bundled onto a stretcher and raced to the nearest Trauma Centre was countered by the experiences of Medicos from the Vietnam War.
Seriously injured casualties had been successfully salvaged by the initiation of intravenous infusion with the fluid bag placed under the casualties shoulder to provide positive pressure during transport by helicopter.

1975 April – Supt. McDonald attended Stage II Ambulance Training School Advanced Paramedical Course

PART TWO with chronological context: THE GOAL POSTS ARE RAISED.

- 1975 Sept. - IAO(Aust.) Proposed Syllabus of knowledge and skills of a Qualified Ambulance Officer – this was the level required to provide BLS to the patient.
- 1975 December - First Seminar in Qld. on Pre-hospital Emergency Patient-care organised and conducted by Mc Donald. The theme "Ambulance – a Broadening Field,"– the topics = Pre-hospital Coronary care and Infusion at scene.
  The then Chairman of the Queensland Division of the Institute, also President of the Superintendent's Association, and the then secretary of the I.A.O. Aust., were not in favour of the Education Seminar nor the topic.
- Participation in State and National development of syllabus for education and assessment of a qualified Ambulance officer – Malcolm submitted items and suggestions to the National body. The original syllabus was examined and amended to 'What the current Ambulance officer could be taught' – there was little changed.
- March 1976 – development of the Training programme for a Qualified Ambulance Officer. M.C. McDonald submitted observations and opinion on this to the National body - . papers available
- July 1976 – even though a Founder member he sat for the examination for elevation from Associate to Member of the Institute using Syllabus subjects
- Nov. 1976 – M.C. McDonald passed the examination on Syllabus subjects as a confirmation of his Founder Member status – this gave him a National qualification and integrity as to his statements.

DIARY : I realised that diary notes were an important part of administration for :-

- Record of appointments to plan schedules
- Record of Superintendents time as he was 'on-call' 24 /7 and had no rostered shifts.
- Record of specific actions/events/directions issued.
- Notes on staff performance and effect of procedures.
- Record of phone instructions from State Council and others as there was great danger of being misquoted or of a denial on what was thought to be of mutual understanding.
- It became a 'ready reference' for the above.

So I kept same at an increasing degree of detail.

My practice of record keeping became well known and my diaries gained a value above worth.

Minister for Health the Hon. Lew Edwards visited Ipswich and inspected Training procedures and the Ambulance Emergency Unit and discussed the Gatton proposal for A/Os to operate a Cardiac monitoring machine on any possible cardiac patient for Doctors information – Dr. Edwards was supportive of this.

1978 April – The Council of the Institute of Ambulance Officers (Aust.) suggests Divisions follow the example of Victoria who have contracted Education Authorities and started a Course using the Institute Syllabus

1978 Sept – I.A.O.(AUST.) Council minutes = NEC has met 3 times

1978 August 1st – Capt. Michael F. Olsen, Senior Medical Services Officer, Medic 1, 301-2nd Ave. SO. Seattle WA.98104 was visiting Australian State Ambulance Services with accommodation at the Gateway Inn, Brisbane.
The State Council / Health Dept. had discouraged him from speaking publically about Advanced Life Support techniques and Procedures in America BUT a couple of we Institute members called on him from 8 pm. and had a good chat, which was quite revealing.

1979 July – Superintendent Mc Donald successfully attended the QASB Ambulance Training School to gain Stage III Certification.

There was still opposition to the curriculum of Training School Courses by Committee and Board members of the QATB as they were in denial of the past practices of Committees.
On a visit to Gatton Centre, QATB State Council member Gerald Moore said he could not appreciate the need for Ambulance officers taking patient observations at scene for submission to a Casualty Dept Doctor 30 minutes or more later!

1979 IPSWICH – I was aware that the Ipswich Superintendent was to retire in a couple of years, here was an opportunity, so I worked to establish my credentials with the Ipswich Committee and in November 1979 I was appointed Superintendent of QATB Ipswich and District.

Ipswich district had :–

- a Regional teaching Hospital;
- a large population = emergencies;
- available financial base;
- sufficient staff.

Now was the opportunity to put into practice and affect my philosophy and direction for the administration of Advanced Life Support for Pre-hospital Emergency patient care by qualified Ambulance officers.
The implementation of any strategy had to provide:-

(1) The education and Certification of officers.
(2) Recording of actual trauma cases treated to prove the procedures were acceptable and the outcomes beneficial to the patient and the Health Dept.
(3) Total commitment for the implementation of this, which would compute to entrenched Medicos, as a radical intervention.

THE EDUCATION OF OFFICERS IN ADVANCED LIFE SUPPORT:

IMMEDIATE : On taking up duties at Ipswich Centre in November of 1979 I established my position as Superintendent and identified the roles and responsibilities of both the administrative staff , the Deputy Superintendent, Station Officers and Ambulance staff.

I was satisfied that the Centre could continue with minimum Managerial supervision so I looked to the core responsibilities of the Centre, that of delivering the highest standard of Pre-hospital Care and set objectives and developed strategies to provide Emergency treatment and Pre-hospital care to National standards within five years for the Ipswich community.
Any Pre-hospital Care system has to be a harmonious co-operation between all members of the Health Care team.

I commenced the training of my Officers in Pre-hospital Emergency Care by attending most Emergency cases and instructing by example, reinforced by 'talks' with demonstrations of techniques and appliances for that specific case.
Each week night Duty officers received instruction on Emergency Care with talks and demonstration of skills and techniques.
Demonstrations of a correctly applied basic Thomas splint was as against a wooden splint each side of the fractured leg, [like stuffing it in a shoebox], supported by blackboard diagrams showing how extension aligned the fractured bones and also the large blood vessels thus controlling haemorrhage and preventing further injury convinced even the most conformist of the superior advantages of the Thomas splint as against conventional wooded splints.

In December 1979 I made an appointment with the IGH Medical Superintendent, Dr. Terry Mulhearn to discuss Hospital and Ambulance objectives.

These addressed the need for local Ambulance Officers to receive basic training in the recognition of patient's respiration patterns and basic airway management, and especially training in the taking of patient's observations to coordinate with Hospital staff recordings as this was a problem area when Officers radioed in with a Report on their patient providing their signs and symptoms – at that period the standard was basic life support.

(A.) Dr. Mulhearn agreed with my policy and the need for training and gave his permission and support by initiating the involvement of Margaret Macfarlane, Director of Nursing who directed Post Operative instruction be organised by Theatre Charge Sister McNulty and RN John Vogel to arrange for Ipswich Officers to attend in Post Operative ward for instruction in taking and recording patient observations.

He also directed me to Dr. Sue Bedford, Intensive Care Consultant, who was most supportive of Ambulance Officers attending in Theatre under supervision (I attended with every officer) for basic airway management instruction.

The support offered by the Chief Executive Officers of Medical/Surgical, Intensive Care and Nursing to my proposed In-hospital Education of Ambulance Officers was total and unconditional - I appreciated their trust.

The Casualty Department was staffed by junior Medical officers up to 1980 and to overcome this problem General Practitioners were employed and it was not till the resolve by Casualty Registrars in the formation of an Association and the conduct of Seminars that positions for Director Emergency Medicine and Outpatient Department was established in 1984. ref: p.149,The Ipswich Hospital 1860-1991.

1980. Jan.11 – Dr. Sue Bedford, IGH Intensive Care Consultant and specialist anaesthetist supported my policy on the overall training of A/O's and for In-theatre training in airway management and advanced skills.
Our discussion concluded with arrangements for staff instruction to commence with the Superintendent attending at IGH Theatre, with single officers in rotation.
The Superintendent to draw up a roster with procedures for Pre- theatre asepsis and gowning etc, and study of Airway management prior to attendance.

(A.1.) In Theatre Training IGH Jan 14th 1980.

- airway management/ resuscitation /shock
- Recovery = patient Observation Report etc. [diary entries]

The In-theatre Airway management program was initiated and the Superintendent attended each Tuesday at Ipswich Regional Hospital theatre section with an Ambulance officer.
This was solely for Airway management – the recognition of breathing patterns – chest movement – insertion of artificial airways – positioning of face mask and procedure for "bagging" the patient and required pressure for inflation of the chest – observation of artificial breathing apparatus – observation of intubation and instruction on cricoid pressure – etc.

This continued until every Ipswich Ambulance Officer had attended on a voluntary basis. This was followed by attendance in Theatre Recovery under instruction of Charge RN McNulty and RN. John Vogel.
Officers took observations of the patient and entered these on the respective forms – officers quickly learned the medical terminology and description of the signs and symptoms of patients with <u>the result of common communication between Hospital and Ambulance staff.</u>

(A.1.ii) The second session for In-theatre training was especially for Senior Officers who had attended the Airway Management and Patient observations instruction as a refresher of that instruction and advanced to patient Resuscitation for fluid replacement and assisting in intubation.

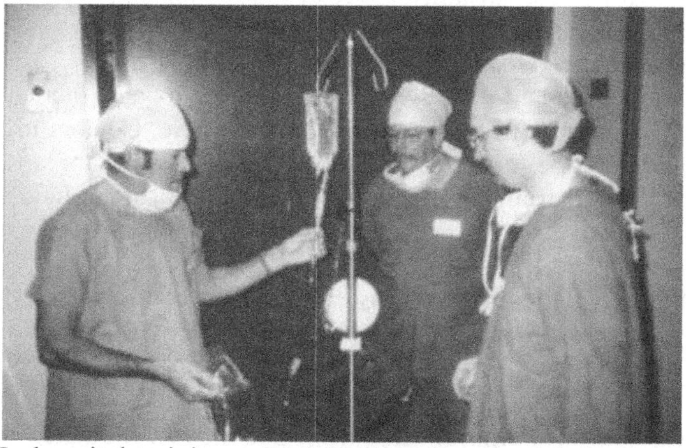

In hospital training – SAO Hall setting up a giving set and adjusting the flow rate, Anaesthetist Dr. S. Page and Supt. McDonald.

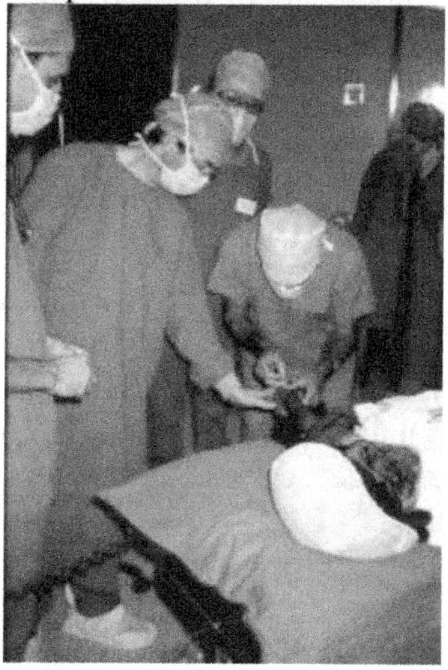

(A.1.ii) cannulation: The second level of In-theatre Training for SAOs.
Drs R. Pascoe &S. Paige, Supt. McDonald, SAO J. Hall.

The QATB Ipswich Committee were well aware of the time I was investing in the upgrading of procedures and staff training at centre and accepted the Training program I had initiated with Medical Superintendent Mulhearn at IGH so it then was a responsible step to propose a Specialised Unit for the regular transfer of Intensive

Care and Surgical patients under Doctor escort from Ipswich to Princess Alexandra and Royal Brisbane Hospitals.

I proposed using one of the single stretcher transport units but to upgrade the equipment for possible emergencies during transport.

(A.2.) On 15th February 1980 we installed specialised equipment in one Ambulance unit for specific patients/casualties. DR. Bedford would accompany intensive care patients being transferred to Brisbane CC or Spinal Units.
Resuscitation equipment of Oxy Viva and Air Viva, aspiration units, oxygen therapy gear, transfusion kits, S.P.P.S. and Haemacell fluids, Entonox, also a "Doctors use ONLY kit" containing, Laryngoscope, endotracheal tubes, Spencer-wells forceps, 'liquorice stick', connector, syringes, cannulas etc, bought from Trust account funds, as done previously in Gatton Units.

This was the first part of the strategy to introduce fully equipped, air conditioned Units to support the future administration of Advanced Life Support by qualified Ambulance officers.

(A.2.i) Feb. 1980 – Accident Report Form [updated from Gatton] was circulated for use on all accident/emergency cases.
This would be was the source document of relevant information:
a. prompt on primary and secondary assessment.
b. recording of trauma cases attended & treatment administered.
c. time frames of callout, at scene and at Hospital.
For retrospective analysis for use in assessment of procedures and treatments to develop a high standard of patient care.

1980 Feb. 15: equipment in Ambulance unit for specialised patients and casualties:
Resuscitation equipment of Oxy Viva and Air Viva, aspiration units, oxygen therapy gear, transfusion kits, S.P.P.S. and Haemacell fluids, Entonox, also a "Doctors use ONLY kit" containing, Laryngoscope, endotracheal tubes, Spencer-wells forceps, 'liquorice stick', connector, syringes, cannulas etc.

This was the strategy to introduce fully equipped, air conditioned Units to support the future administration of Advanced Life Support by qualified Ambulance officers.

Nothing was without risk when one pushes the implementing of new equipment and innovative procedures:
I went close to dismissal for this initiative as I had pushed the Committee to accept my proposal and innovations.
The one being air conditioning which was opposed by a couple of the Committee.
When I took them for a demo - THE AIR CON DID NOT WORK.

I suffered much castigation and had sleepless nights before I took it out of the hands of Superior Body Builders and was able to correct and fix it through the Ipswich Air Conditioning firm.
Negative comment oft stated:

PRESS REPORT: 1980 February-
State Council Vice Chair " a little knowledge could be a dangerous thing."

This statement was often spoken by the Health Dept. Medical Officer as a control of any progressive move as a perceived invasion into the realm of the Medical officer.
ref: Courier Mail press cutting.

Queensland Times 25.3.1980:

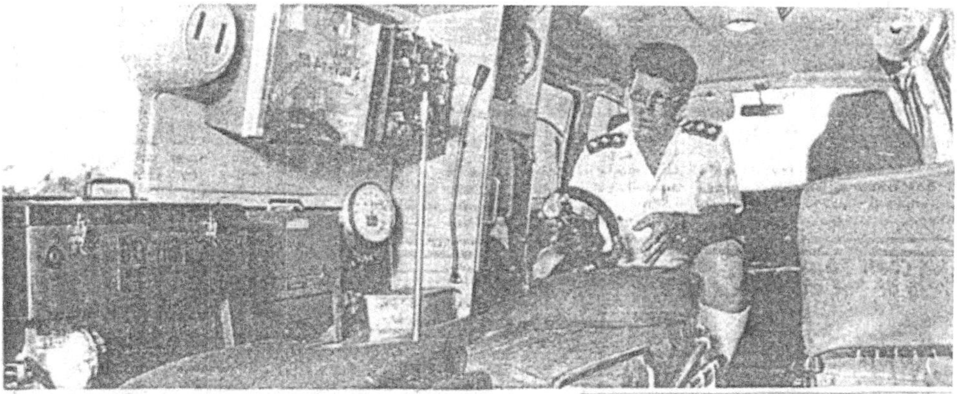

QATB Ipswich centre superintendent, Mr M. C. McDonald is pictured in the "doctor's seat" of the new special care ambulance recently commissioned by the centre.

Equipment carried in the "Special Care Unit" IPSWICH 1980

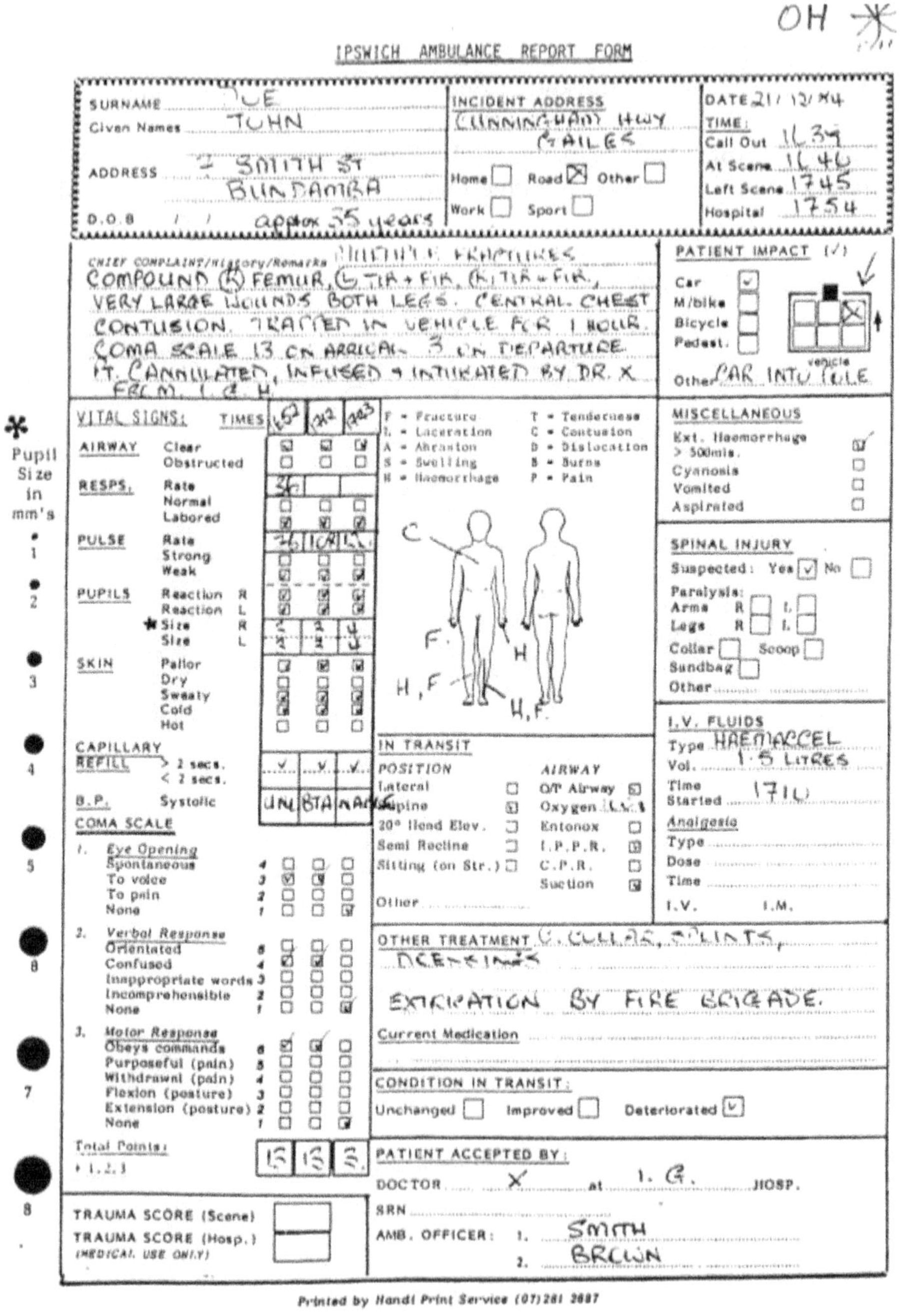

OH *

IPSWICH AMBULANCE REPORT FORM

SURNAME DUE
Given Names JOHN
ADDRESS 2 SMITH ST BUNDAMBA
D.O.B / / approx 35 years

INCIDENT ADDRESS CUNNINGHAM HWY GAILES
Home ☐ Road ☒ Other ☐
Work ☐ Sport ☐

DATE 21/12/84
TIME:
Call Out 1639
At Scene 1646
Left Scene 1745
Hospital 1754

CHIEF COMPLAINT/History/Remarks MULTIPLE FRACTURES
COMPOUND (R) FEMUR, (L) TIB + FIB, (R) TIB + FIB,
VERY LARGE WOUNDS BOTH LEGS. CENTRAL CHEST
CONTUSION. TRAPPED IN VEHICLE FOR 1 HOUR.
COMA SCALE 13 ON ARRIVAL 3 ON DEPARTURE.
PT. CANNULATED, INFUSED + INTUBATED BY DR. X
FRCM. I.G.H.

PATIENT IMPACT (✓)
Car ☑
M/bike ☐
Bicycle ☐
Pedest. ☐
Other CAR INTO vehicle TRUCK

VITAL SIGNS:		TIMES	1652	1712	1743
AIRWAY	Clear		☑	☑	☑
	Obstructed		☐	☐	☐
RESPS.	Rate		36		
	Normal		☐	☐	☐
	Labored		☑	☑	☑
PULSE	Rate		136	140	146
	Strong		☐	☐	☐
	Weak		☑	☑	☑
PUPILS	Reaction	R	☑	☑	☑
	Reaction	L	☑	☑	☑
	* Size	R	2	3	4
	Size	L	2	3	4
SKIN	Pallor		☑	☑	☑
	Dry		☐	☐	☐
	Sweaty		☑	☑	☑
	Cold		☑	☑	☑
	Hot		☐	☐	☐
CAPILLARY REFILL	> 2 secs.		✓	✓	✓
	< 2 secs.				
B.P.	Systolic		UN	OBTA	INABLE

COMA SCALE

1. Eye Opening	Spontaneous	4	☐	☐	☐
	To voice	3	☑	☑	☐
	To pain	2	☐	☐	☐
	None	1	☐	☐	☑
2. Verbal Response	Orientated	5	☐	☐	☐
	Confused	4	☑	☑	☐
	Inappropriate words	3	☐	☐	☐
	Incomprehensible	2	☐	☐	☐
	None	1	☐	☐	☑
3. Motor Response	Obeys commands	6	☑	☑	☐
	Purposeful (pain)	5	☐	☐	☐
	Withdrawal (pain)	4	☐	☐	☐
	Flexion (posture)	3	☐	☐	☐
	Extension (posture)	2	☐	☐	☐
	None	1	☐	☐	☑
Total Points: 1.2.3			13	13	3

* Pupil Size in mm's: 1, 2, 3, 4, 5, 6, 7, 8

F - Fracture, L - Laceration, A - Abrasion, S - Swelling, H - Haemorrhage, T - Tenderness, C - Contusion, D - Dislocation, B - Burns, P - Pain

C, F, H, H,F, H,F

MISCELLANEOUS
Ext. Haemorrhage > 500mls. ☑
Cyanosis ☐
Vomited ☐
Aspirated ☐

SPINAL INJURY
Suspected: Yes ☑ No ☐
Paralysis:
Arms R ☐ L ☐
Legs R ☐ L ☐
Collar ☐ Scoop ☐
Sandbag ☐
Other

I.V. FLUIDS
Type HAEMACCEL
Vol. 1.5 LITRES
Time Started 1710
Analgesia
Type
Dose
Time
I.V. I.M.

IN TRANSIT
POSITION
Lateral ☐
Supine ☑
20° Head Elev. ☐
Semi Recline ☐
Sitting (on Str.) ☐
Other

AIRWAY
O/P Airway ☑
Oxygen 10 L
Entonox ☐
I.P.P.R. ☑
C.P.R. ☐
Suction ☑

OTHER TREATMENT C. COLLAR, SPLINTS, DRESSINGS
EXTRICATION BY FIRE BRIGADE.
Current Medication

CONDITION IN TRANSIT:
Unchanged ☐ Improved ☐ Deteriorated ☑

PATIENT ACCEPTED BY:
DOCTOR X at I. G. HOSP.
SRN
AMB. OFFICER: 1. SMITH
2. BROWN

TRAUMA SCORE (Scene)
TRAUMA SCORE (Hosp.)
(MEDICAL USE ONLY)

Printed by Handi Print Service (07) 281 2887

IPSWICH ambulance Report form 1984.

Following page:-
SCHEMATIC DIAGRAM of the role of Services and Officers at a major Emergency -

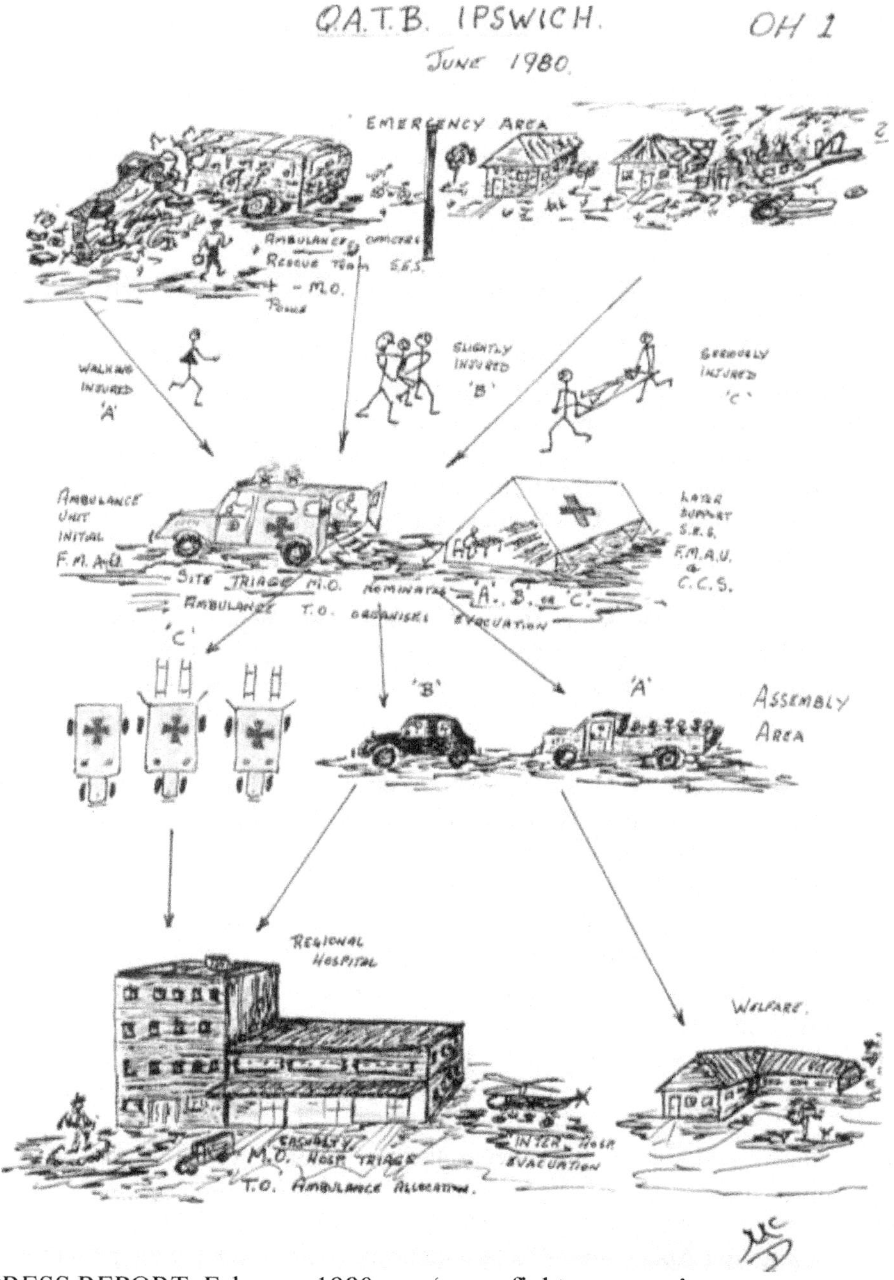

PRESS REPORT: February 1980: 'some fight progress.'
State Council Vice Chair " a little knowledge could be a dangerous thing."
This statement was often spoken by the Health Dept. Medical Officer.
Courier Mail press cutting.
NOTE: All Training at Ipswich was documented as was the assessments with signing off by the Doctor, the Charge Sister and the Officer.

1980: TRAINING WAS 'STEP BY STEP' - towards professionalism.

Supt. McDonald attended cases as the 1st Officer and the AO on duty acted as assistant, so initial training was by example and hands on.
This was followed up by a discussion on all aspects of the case and on return to Centre by whiteboard and equipment 'talk.'
As Officers received this education, they realized what they didn't know and wanted to learn more.
Super compiled Study sheets and conducted training 'sessions' almost daily.

As Chairman of the Qld. Division of the Institute of Ambulance Officers (Aust.) I used this position to convince anyone and everyone [Officers, Health Dept. Medicos, State Council, etc.] that Advanced Pre-hospital Emergency Care was the acceptable norm and to give the Ambulance Officers a belief in themselves - every talk, address, paper, presentation mentioned the professionalism of officers.
BUT, if we were to introduce ALS training we had to also include recognition by position/pay structure.

Each Minister for Health was kept informed of Seminars and the Topics discussed and Department of Health Officers were invited to functions at Centre where the Training facilities, equipment and Units of the Centre would be shown to effect. Doctors Donaldson and Kemp.

The QATB structure gave the ideal employment environment to introduce different levels of qualifications on a pass/fail assessment without disadvantaging employees as to the wage rate they were receiving.
QATB already had different levels of employment:-

- Transport Officer – basic qualifications only for patient transports.
- Ambulance Officer – basic qualifications, plus QATB Training School stages.
- Senior Ambulance Officer – Ambulance Officer with min of 3 years service generally limited to one or two staff.

This provided the atmosphere for the concept that Senior Officers might be appointed on the basis that they have ALS qualifications .

The State Council could not see this concept; they were satisfied with the status quo.

As a test exercise on March 10th 1980, an Ambulance officer cannulated patient 'In-Theatre' at IGH and on April 14th 1980 the Superintendent intubated the patient in IGH Theatre under the supervision of the Consultant. diary note
PROOF POSITIVE THAT QLD. AMBULANCE OFFICERS ARE CAPABLE OF BEING TRAINED IN ADVANCED LIFE SUPPORT –
In-theatre training of Ambulance officers continued for airway management and patient observation for officers until all staff had attended.

ADVANCED TRAINING FOR STAGE 1 OFFICERS:

On the completion of the first round of In-theatre training, Stage 1 officers with over three years experience, (as a control measure), were instructed in intravenous cannulation of the patient and to assist the Medical officer with intubation of the patient at scene.

Dr. Sue Bedford had set the tone and progressive standard for the In-theatre training for Ipswich Ambulance Officers, and after she left IGH, the education of officers continued under the Director of Anaesthetics Ranald Pascoe, and Drs S. Paige, L. Coaldrake, as well as Private Drs M. Cobcroft and others.

I am most appreciative of the support I received from Dr. Bedford and the bond formed on the provision of 'best practice' in all Ambulance procedures.

June 1980 – Superintendent McDonald presented a paper "Problems of Evacuation and Transportation" at a Qld. Accident & Emergency Association Conference.

THE INSTITUTE IS THE KEY, it gave the venue and the platform for education for Ambulance Officers.

Only officers interested in education/training joined the Institute and attended seminars – it was not an industrial association/union – of course there were a couple of exceptions: (1) to keep control, and (2) the 'foot in each camp' nonentity.

1981 January – paper on "Rescue in the Ambulance Service" Institute Seminar at Gatton College

1982 May - Course Comparisons between QATB Training School and the Institute Course referred to Bundaberg Workshop closing address by the Chair IAO Qld. M.C. McDonald 16.5.1982. [p. 25 in IAO Membership course folder]

McDonald compiled booklets for study from those of the 17 Units not covered by QATB Training School. The content for study and assessment was the important aspect not how the study booklets were published. NB. copies available.

1982. **(A.3),** QATB Ipswich now has officers certified for (IV) cannulation and infusion therapy and assisting with Intubation.

1983 June – Supt. McDonald attended Ambulance Training School Stage III Refresher course.

On receiving his Certification for successfully passing this Course, the Superintendent compiled a syllabus for a TRAINING VIDEO ON ADVANCED LIFE SUPPORT for potential Senior Officers at Ipswich.

ADVANCED TRAINING BY VIDEO, JUNE 1983.

The Superintendent was assisted by Deputy Supt. Bob Watson and Station Officer John Hall with Officer Alan Feldon as the Video producer.

A.L.S. TRAINING AT IPSWICH 1983:

Selection of Staff Training photos from frames of original Video Training tape.

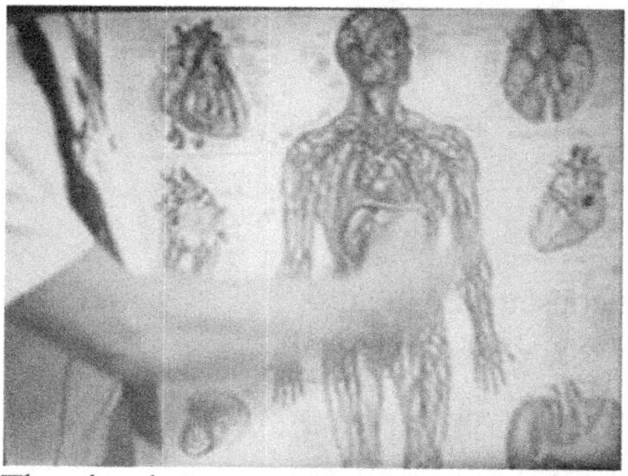

The circulatory system and vital organs, relative to injury and blood loss.

RESUSCITATION:

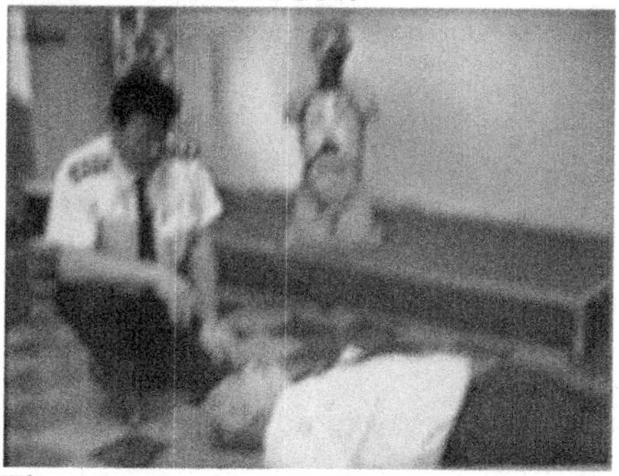

The unconscious patient.

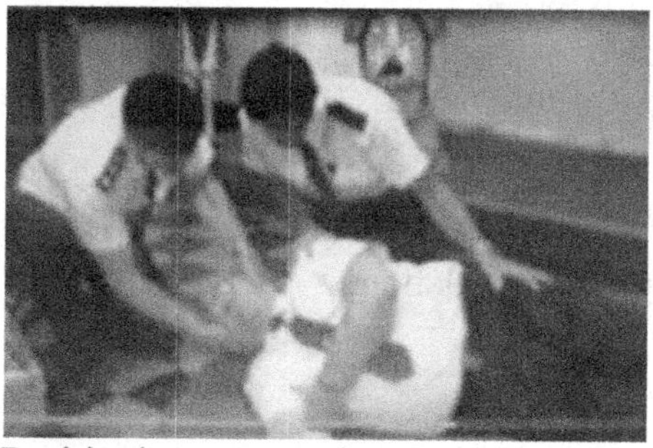

Positioning unconscious patient – protection of the cervical spine.

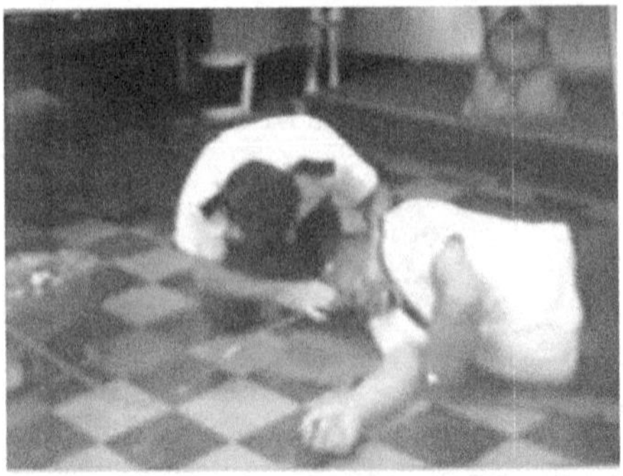

Aspiration of the unconscious patient –
using suction from Oxy Viva- SO J. Hall.

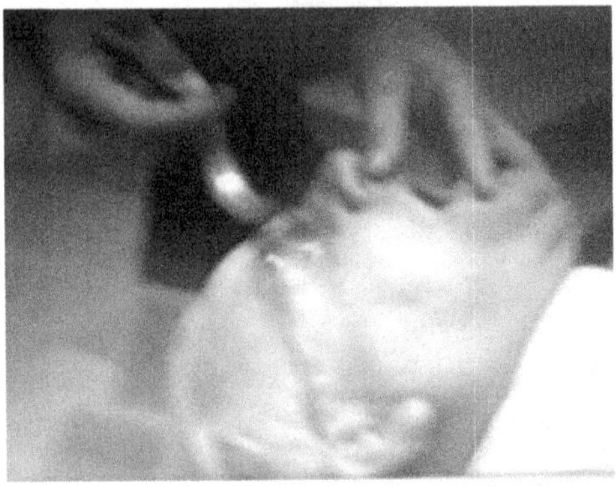

Supt. inserting artificial airway in the unconscious patient

PAEDRIATRIC RESUS.

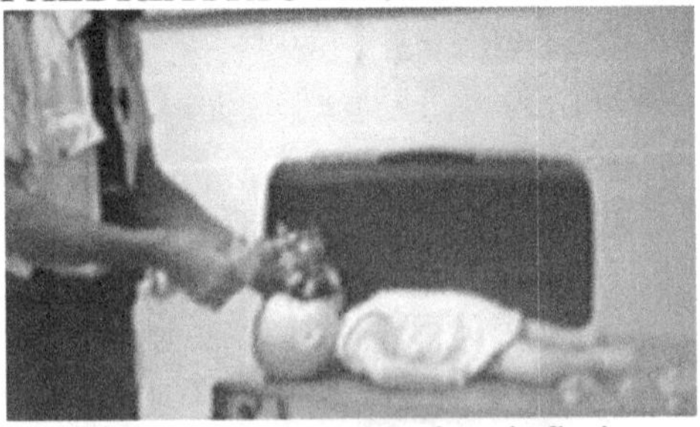

Positioning of airway before inflation.

INTRAVENOUS INFUSION TECHNIQUES
as videoed for staff training:

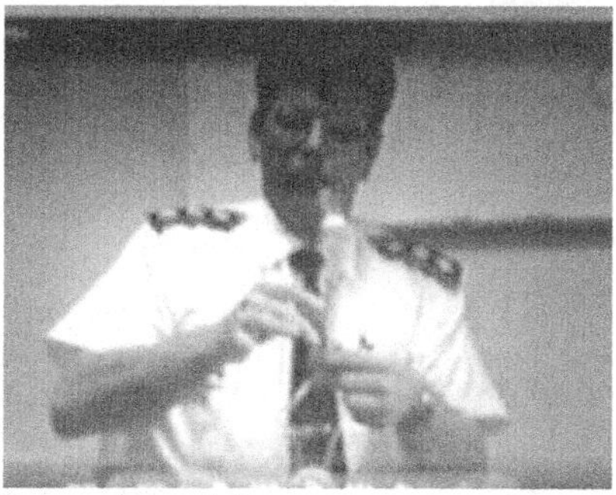

Preparing giving set.

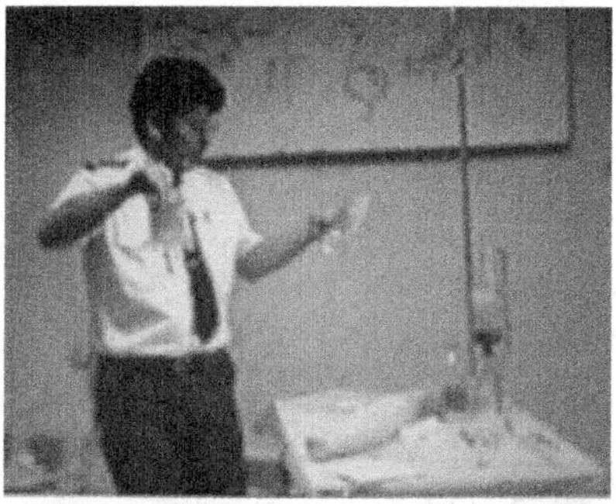

Different fluids and different size bags

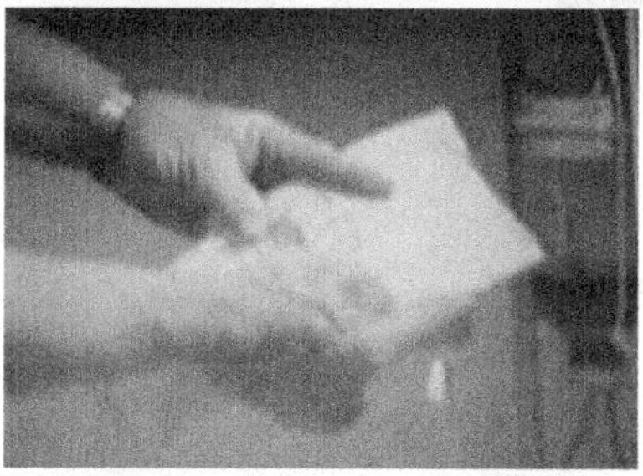

Double check for correct fluid and the expiry date.

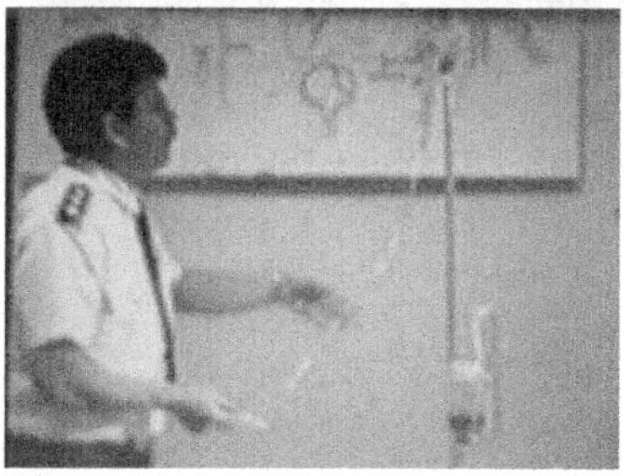

First run of fluid to remove air bubbles

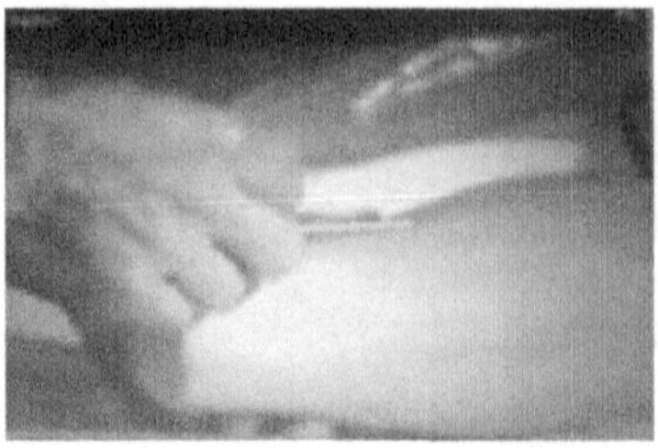

Inserting cannula – bevel up, beside vein before entering vein.

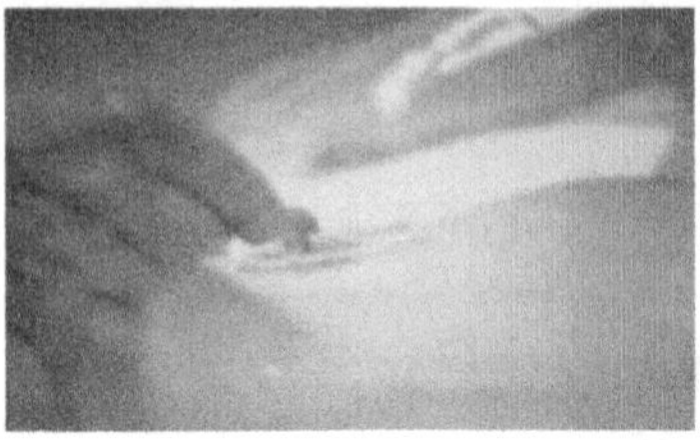

On insertion of cannula check for flash back of blood before
partly withdrawing the metal trocar and further introducing the Teflon catheter.

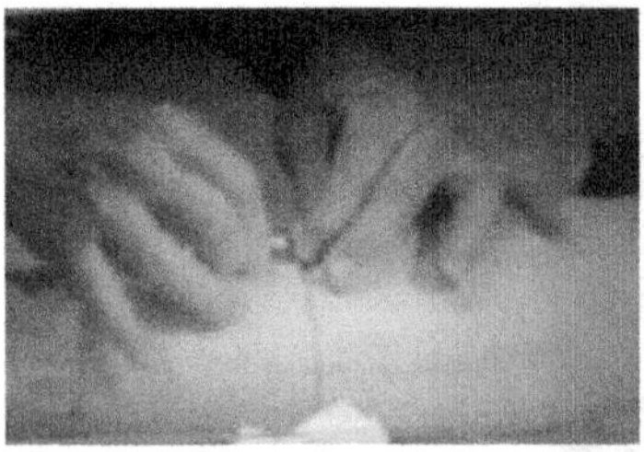

Inserting giving set into catheter insitu.

The catheter is then anchored to the arm by firstly a ½ inch wide strip of adhesive tape applied to the arm, under the catheter, then taken over the catheter, then under to cross over the initial tape, thus anchoring the catheter securely in place.
A specific transparent dressing can then be applied over the junction of the tube with the catheter.

FRACTURES WHICH CAUSE FLOOD LOSS.

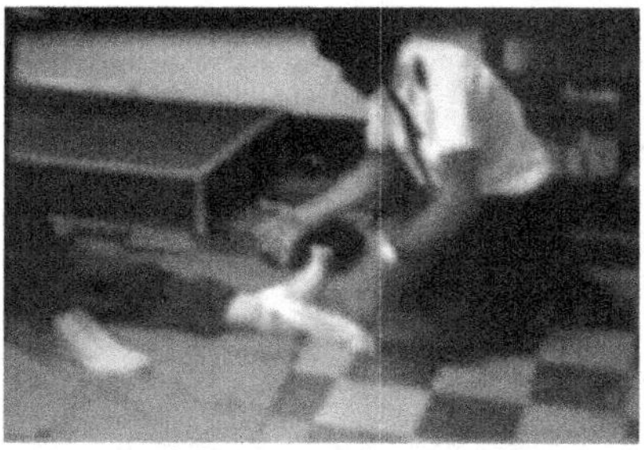
Fractured femur: SO. J. Hall, preparing for application of Thomas splint – bottle knot.

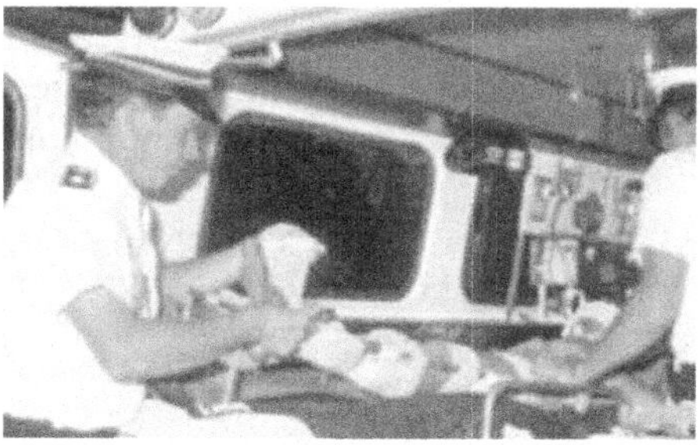
Thomas splint for fractured femur.

QATB Ipswich now had a number of Officers with the capability to administer ALS and intravenous infusion at scene on telephonic permission.
1983 – Ipswich Committee appoints Senior Ambulance Officers by demonstration of knowledge and skills and rosters a Senior Ambulance Officer as the first officer supported by a second Officer on the Emergency Unit on each shift of the 24 hours.
With the support of the Ipswich Committee I now have the certified ambulance officer levels and the comparative pay structure which supports the added skills of :-

- Senior Ambulance officer – qualifications to levels of Advanced Life Support of Pre-hospital Emergency Care = 1st officer

The 1st Officer received a wage allowance as a 'Senior Officer.'
It was up to the Union now to support Education and Qualifications and to seek comparative wage rates.

THIS WAS THE TURNING POINT – this proved Ambulance Officers could be trained in Advanced Life Support techniques and be assessed with a PASS/ FAIL. This was tested by Union examination and also by an unsuccessful court Appeal by one officer.
NB: An Ipswich staff member on the State Union executive was always present and I always discussed any innovation in a positive manner with him and received his support.

The State Council should have introduced this years ago.
NOTE: Education and training in Advanced Life Support techniques continued for Ipswich officers.
Qualified officers carried out intravenous cannulation at scene with either permission from the IGH Casualty Dept or from a Doctor at scene.

This was recorded on case sheets and Accident Report Forms.
Retrospective analysis was carried out on Accident Report Forms and these findings were discussed with officers by STO Tony Reader.

It was not until 1987 when Ipswich was able to run computerised analysis.

A reporting program for stats of type and time was developed and run on the Centre computer using the Call sheets and accident Report Forms as source documents. 1987, ref P&P 75a– this gave quality control and a visible analysis of results.

COMPUTERISED RECORDS OF CASES ATTENDED & STATS.

Ipswich Computer stats 1987 75a
for analysis of particular category within 24 hours.

Q.A.T.B. (IPSWICH).
CASELOAD x CATEGORY x TIME PERIODS

30-06-87
Page 2

Report for Month of May
for Branch IPSWICH

CATEGORY	0-2	2-4	4-6	6-8	8-10	10-12	12-14	14-16	16-18	18-20	20-22	22-24	INVAL	TOTAL
ROAD ACCIDENT														
Cases	4	0	0	3	0	6	2	4	6	1	4	1	0	31
Hours	1.72	0.00	0.00	1.99	0.00	1.81	0.15	1.52	3.10	1.00	1.70	0.98	0.00	[illegible]
Klms	67	0	0	44	0	28	5	18	52	5	17	10	14	260
CHEST PAINS														
Cases	2	1	0	3	3	4	7	5	3	3	2	3	0	36
Hours	1.73	0.78	0.00	2.27	2.87	2.84	4.64	4.07	3.82	2.59	1.13	2.99	0.00	[illegible]
Klms	15	16	0	25	32	37	46	61	88	31	17	51	0	419
URGENT MEDICAL														
Cases	3	3	1	9	21	15	14	12	8	8	8	10	0	112
Hours	2.72	2.65	0.85	7.02	14.74	10.35	8.62	8.67	6.87	6.87	5.24	6.27	0.00	80.67
Klms	47	47	11	138	219	173	227	98	184	145	76	133	0	1496
OTHER														
Cases	0	0	0	8	19	21	8	21	21	6	8	6	7	125
Hours	0.00	0.00	0.00	20.96	42.34	52.28	4.73	13.94	3.41	1.83	26.93	2.17	0.00	168.53
Klms	0	0	0	101	154	166	77	177	72	23	62	54	52	938
RESUSITATION														
Cases	0	0	0	0	1	0	0	0	0	0	0	0	0	1
Hours	0.00	0.00	0.00	0.00	0.73	0.00	0.00	0.00	0.00	0.00	0.00	0.00	0.00	0.73
Klms	0	0	0	0	8	0	0	0	0	0	0	0	0	8
URGENT SURGICAL														
Cases	0	0	0	1	0	1	0	0	0	0	0	0	0	2
Hours	0.00	0.00	0.00	0.72	0.00	0.35	0.00	0.00	0.00	0.00	0.00	0.00	0.00	1.07
Klms	0	0	0	7	0	8	0	0	0	0	0	0	0	15
TRAUMA														
Cases	4	0	1	4	6	5	10	15	10	6	3	3	0	57
Hours	2.61	0.00	1.13	2.01	3.00	4.25	5.69	12.00	8.17	4.57	0.97	2.88	0.00	47.38
Klms	37	0	23	35	38	75	102	241	174	105	16	39	26	911
WHITE														
Cases	6	3	5	319	269	318	273	201	82	23	24	10	18	[illegible]
Hours	5.62	3.15	2.27	277.90	115.98	145.29	158.31	104.41	40.92	16.30	19.04	5.21	0.00	[illegible]
Klms	199	93	78	3644	2803	3405	3789	2516	986	335	500	125	334	[illegible]
TOTAL CASES	19	7	7	347	319	370	314	258	130	47	49	33	25	1925
TOTAL HRS.	14.42	6.58	4.25	312.87	173.66	217.17	182.14	144.6[illegible]	65.49	33.26	55.0[illegible]	20.42	0.00	1235.86
TOTAL KLMS	365	156	112	3994	3254	3892	4246	3113	1558	704	688	412	426	22927

MINES RESCUE DEPOT – 22 Aug.1987 - gas cylinder explosion.

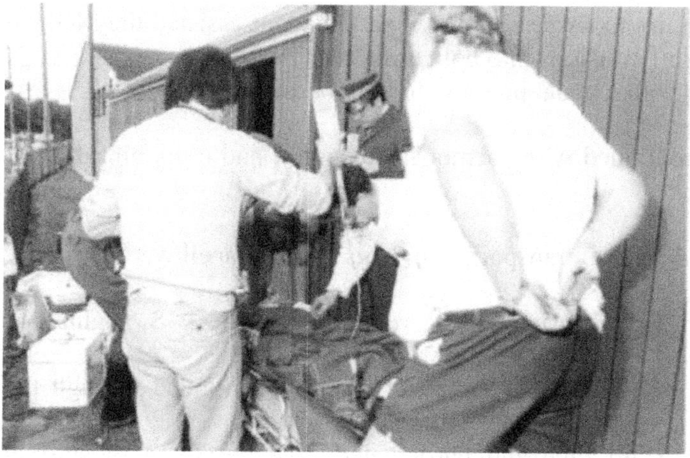

Whilst checking equipment the Superintendent of the Mines Rescue Station, Ipswich suffered serious injury when an explosion occurred whilst he was working with a 2 ½ litre cylinder of methane gas.

As Mines Rescue had a strong reputation for Safety procedures there had to be unusual circumstance for this to occur -
Mines Rescue used oxygen and methane gas for Training Instruction and cylinders were sent to BOC for refilling but inexplicably a cylinder with oxygen had been toped up with methane and delivered.
On BOC realising their error, they informed the Mines Rescue Superintendent of the situation, identified the cylinder and advised the need to return it urgently.

The Mines Rescue Superintendent now had a potential "bomb" and didn't want to drive it in the car, so negotiated to go to a local open cut to bury it.
Even this was risky so he decided to open it and decant the gas under water in a large bin but he was unable to get the valve open.

By this he was under a degree of stress and to obtain a firmer grip on the valve he removed the cylinder from the water and placed it on the grass beside the Training Gallery and opened it carefully – there was an instantaneous flash and explosion.
ref: Mines Rescue member.

He suffered multiple fractures to on his left side from hip to foot with extensive tissue damage.
On arrival the Ambulance Officers diagnosed hypovolemic shock and that any movement would cause greater blood loss – they radioed for Medical assistance at scene.

As per MOP protocol Supt. McDonald collected the Senior A and E Medical Officer from IGH and on arrival at scene an infusion of SPPS was immediately administered to the leg to maintain viability to tissue and the Superintendent assisted the Medical officer to 'put up' Haemacell infusions into both arms of the patient.
These were run fully open with manual pressure to both bags.

The Ambulance officers continued with haemorrhage control and immobilisation of the fractures with splints.

On loading the patient, and prior to transport, both bags of Haemacell were replaced.

The hospital was notified and the Ambulance proceeded with L & S, (lights and siren).
The patient had a positive attitude from the onset and this continued through the fitting of a prosthesis and the following physiotherapy.
He returned to work in record time and participated in the training of staff in underground procedures.

Doug set a highly respected officer of the Mines Rescue Brigade.

ALLEGY – pain relief:

At Ipswich, the Emergency call had come in as an electrocution, so Control had notified me to standby in case a Doctor was required at scene (we did not have defibrillators at that point.)

I was notified that the patient was conscious, but severely burned, and the crew had requested a Doctor for pain relief as per our Protocols.

I arranged to meet Dr. Gerry FitzGerald at the Ipswich hospital, drove him to meet the ambulance unit, left the retrieval car at roadside, and we both returned with the patient, the Doctor to administer any necessary drugs, and myself as extra hands to assist or in case the patient arrested.

The Senior officer gave us a report on the history of the accident and the patient's obs.
The patient had been working on a large industrial switchboard, checking for a fault. He found the fault - **FLASH** - but in so doing had created a short circuit in the wiring, causing an electrical arc with its intense heat and flash of electricity.

The patient suffered superficial and partial thickness burns to his full face and neck, he was approximately 22 years old.
This was causing him *extreme* pain.

Doctor FitzGerald requested that an infusion set be put up -- he cannulated the patient, then requested drugs from the Medical kit which I selected and passed to him repeating the name, he checked, then drew up pain relieving drugs, and asked relevant information from the patient before he administered the I.V. injection.

The patient was groaning, and twisting in pain, on the stretcher.

" Are you **allergic** to anything ? " asked Dr. FitzGerald.

Through gritted teeth the young man replied,
" **ONLY FLASH BURNS, DOC.**"

Yes, it's good to be able to laugh, even if only inwardly.

BUT BUREAUCRACY IS NOTHING TO LAUGH ABOUT
AS THE NEXT ARTICLE DEMONSTRATES

REMOVE ALL HUMIDIFIERS .

I was more than surprised when I received an instruction from the secretary of the QATB State Council that, " all Humidifiers are to removed from Ambulance Units."

I rang Ernie Bradley and asked what this was all about? He told me that a senior Doctor in the Health Department had ruled that 'humidifiers were means of cross infection and were inefficient' and therefore should be removed.

The first thing that came to mind was, "what poppycock" for I had done my research on the value of humidified oxygen for certain cases and especially to patients suffering inhalation of hot air or burning gases, and secondly, any concern of 'cross infection' was no reason to remove equipment, the positive action would be to sterilise the equipment.

I wrote to the State Council stating that I could not accept the reasons for removing Humidifiers, that cross infection could be controlled by sterilisation and that Ipswich would not be removing this equipment from their units unless something better was supplied.

Our problem in administering pre-hospital emergency care was not being permitted, or trained in the use of, sophisticated equipment and procedures for the treatment of emergency conditions.
It behove the Superintendent and the Ambulance officers to use every available technique to alleviate the patient's condition and to assist in their recovery process, *we could not allow for the removal of any one of the technical equipment available to us without fighting to keep it or to gain something better.*

I then started to look into the allegations:-

- I knew that medical oxygen was 'dry.'
- that patients suffering from inhalation of hot air or burning gases had burns to their airway and possibly bronchus which would result in oedema of the tissues.
- it was imperative that cool, moist oxygen was administered as soon as possible to alleviate this condition.
- the only way to achieve this was by the use of oxygen through an humidifier.

The Doctor had said the humidifier was inefficient, well, we had to prove her wrong. Therefore we must test the system.
We'd need a quality instrument to measure humidity, who? where?

I started by asking staff if anyone had a quality weather instrument, one that measured the humidity of the air to indicate rain etc.
I struck pay dirt immediately; Station Officer Jim Smith said he had a relatively new, desk top instrument enclosed in a clear plastic bubble with an aperture at each side – ideal. I asked him to take a car and collect it from his home.

Now for the 'test centre.'

I set up a test site at the side of the plant room floor, [in an area free of oil and grease], a couple of cylinders of medical oxygen with oxygen therapy equipment, tubing, humidifier, tape, humidity instrument and report sheets.

Station Officer Smith and another officer followed my instructions:-

- the reading was taken of the humidity of the air and the time noted, signed off
- the tubing was inserted into one aperture of the instrument and taped in place. The reading was checked again.
- the oxygen was turned on and after a minute or so the reading of the instrument was taken, recorded and signed off. It was actually lower than the ambient air.
- the oxygen was turned off and the humidifier was connected to the oxygen therapy equipment and the bowl filled to the mark with room temperature water.
- another reading was taken of the instrument, recorded with the time and signed off.
- the oxygen was turned on at the 4 l.min flow rate, and bubbled through the humidifier and on through the instrument.
- after a couple of minutes the reading was taken and recorded with the time.

It was observed that the humidified oxygen flowing through the instrument was of higher humidity than the ambient air and much higher humidity to the dry medical oxygen.
One of the Police Sergeants from Ipswich Headquarters happened to call to check with me about some mutual business, so I asked him if he would watch our experiment and then countersign the findings, he was happy to participate.

A second run of further tests of checking the ambient air, then the dry oxygen, then the humidified oxygen, were carried out, with the same results showing that the humidified oxygen was of a higher humidity than both the ambient air and the dry oxygen from the cylinder.
The Sergeant counter signed the new recordings.

We had only finished our experiment and I was actually dictating a letter to State Council regarding same when the phone rang, I answered and the voice said :- "This is Tom Watson, Malcolm," it was Dr. Watson the Medical adviser to State Council, oh dear, what was he about to say ?

"Yes doctor, how can I help you" I answered.

"Malcolm, you are to have all the Humidifiers at the centre and in the units tested by the Pathology section of the Ipswich Hospital, give them a ring and arrange for this to be done when it suits you please."

"Yes Doctor, I'll attend to it straight away," we talked generally for a while then closed the conversation. I believed I had 'got the message.'

I knew Dr. Watson from various meetings and had found him to be dedicated to Pre-hospital Care and easy to approach, I believed he was giving me the opportunity to 'back-up' my statement regarding "all Humidifiers are to removed from Ambulance Units."

I thought for a while then dictated to my secretary an Official Notice to staff, to be typed immediately for distribution.

Procedure for the use and sterilisation of Humidifiers.
1) after use all humidifiers are to be removed from the unit and replaced from stock.
2) after use all humidifiers are to be dismantled, washed with soap and water and all threaded and jointed areas scrubbed in preparation for sterilisation.
3) all parts to be steam sterilised for min of 20 minutes, then allowed to dry on the steriliser tray.
4) the dry equipment is to be placed in a sterile paper bag, sealed and replaced in stock.

USE.
1) when required the humidifier is to be removed from the sealed bag, the bowl is to be filled to the mark with sterile water from the sealed bags in the unit.
2) the oxygen is to be supplied at the optimum flow rate and administered via disposable mask and tubing.
THIS TO BE EFFECTED IMMEDIATELY.

I had four of these notices typed, met with my Deputy, explained the situation and he then placed these on each of the staff notice boards.
He then organised the removal, in turn, of all the humidifiers from the units and had them sterilised and sealed in sterile bags.

As soon as the first humidifier unit had been sterilised and bagged, I rang Dr. David McAdam Director of Ipswich Pathology, identified myself and explained what I had been instructed.
He answered in his friendly manner and said that he had been informed by Dr.Watson and if we dropped any spare units into the section he would have them checked for contamination and provide a report on completion of all units.
This was done and of course all the units were declared clean and free of any infection.

Presentation to State Council:
I then submitted a full presentation to State Council of the witnessed tests carried out on the Humidifier and the resultant findings in its favour as to its efficiency and thereby its effectiveness.

I drew attention to the Report on the sterility of all Humidifier units and the Procedure in place for the administration of humidified oxygen therapy.
I concluded that I saw no need for the removal of Humidifiers from Ambulance units and in fact suggested that State Council ensure that all Ambulance units throughout the State be stocked with this equipment.

I cannot remember if I received an answer, but there was no further action taken by State Council. A couple of weeks later I did receive a phone call from a Charge Sister of a major Brisbane Public hospital asking me for full particulars of my submission to State Council so that they too could stop removal of this equipment from their Casualty.

Again, if you believe in something then you should take the appropriate steps to keep it or to initiate it, but, always check and double check your facts and ensure that all is certified and correctly applied.

QATB IPSWICH COMMITTEE:
At all times I kept Chairman John Cushing and the Ipswich Committee informed of every aspect of Training I wished to introduce and outlined the professional advancement for officers and the resultant benefit to any member of the community at large.

At all times the Committee supported me and in this and provided any necessary requirement to ensure the end result.

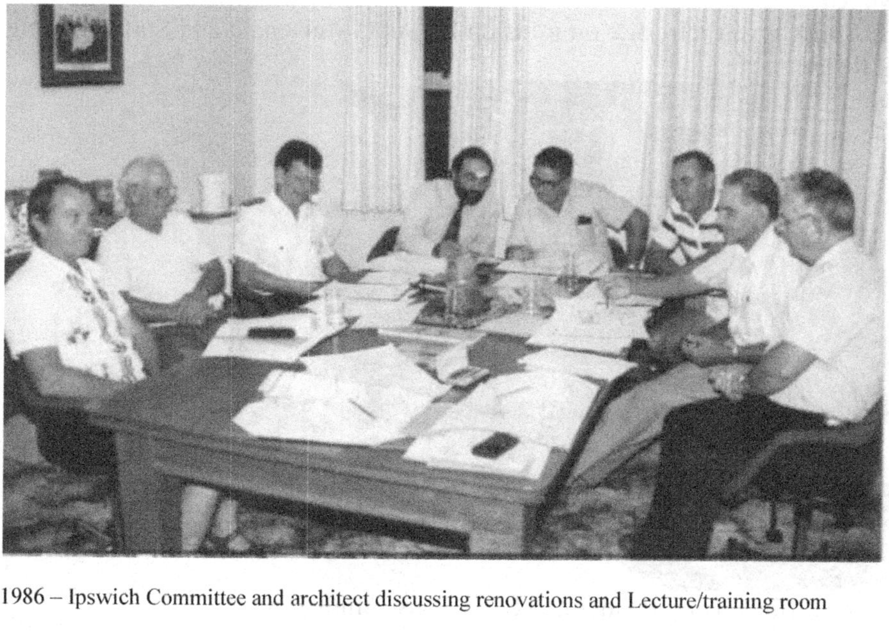

1986 – Ipswich Committee and architect discussing renovations and Lecture/training room

THE FIRST TRAINING OFFICER OUTSIDE THE CTS - the Central Training School.

1983. An increase in the number of staff and the upgraded levels of Training demanded too much of my time to supervise as Superintendent and I recommended to the Ipswich Committee to appoint a staff Training Officer.
So we had to make-up his designation, role and wage structure.

We had Tony Reader as a Senior Officer with responsibility for staff Training. He had certain wage conditions re penalties etc to give an appropriate wage.

NATIONAL PRESIDENT OF IAO(AUST.).
In 1984 M. McDonald was elected the National President of the Institute of Ambulance Officers (Aust.) for a three year term.
The previous and inaugural President had originally been a member of the NSW Ambulance Board.
As President he used every opportunity to present the case for professionalism in Ambulance Officers:

- education
- certification
- Advanced Life Support at scene

1984 presented paper "Trauma and Medical Emergencies" at an Institute Seminar in Rockhampton.

INTRAVENOUS CANNULATION TECHNIQUES :
1984- 6 March:
(1) A/O T. Smith given refresher on infusion by Supt. McDonald and Staff Training Officer T. Reader

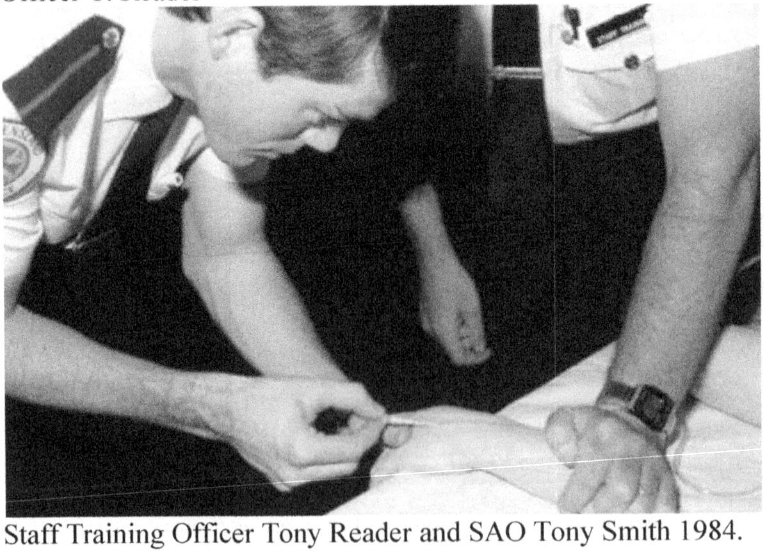

Staff Training Officer Tony Reader and SAO Tony Smith 1984.

(2) Dr. Gerald Fitzgerald examined A/O Hall and qualified him for infusions.
(3) Supt McDonald researching a paper on the premise 'that an infusion is not a drug in the meaning of "the Act."

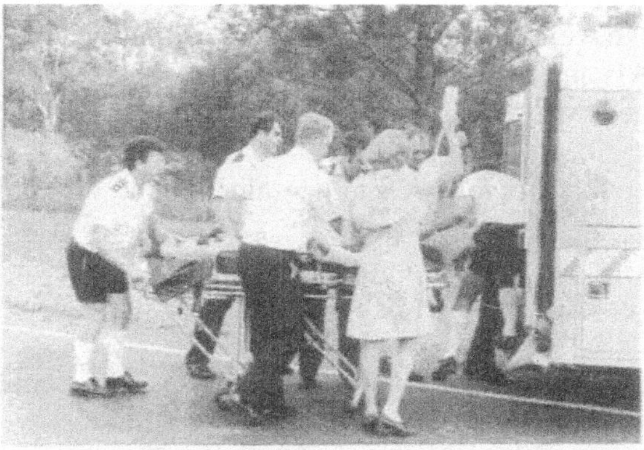

TRAINING PUT INTO PRACTICE - Supt. and TO Reader respond to accident victim requiring fluid replacement 1984.

1984. 22 March: Gailes Railway accident with three casualties from train accident requiring cannulation and infusion by Ambulance officers at scene- D/Supt. John Hall.
IGH Emergency Director Dr. Fitzgerald present. ref. diary entry.

1984.April 8– Road accident: The Senior AO at scene called for Medical assistance so as per protocol. Superintendent collected the medical officer on duty at IGH and proceeded to the incident. Lights and siren, adrenalin flowing.
Reported 'arrival on scene.'
Senior Officer Plotski gave a report on the patient's injuries and that he was in shock and required extrication.
On assessing the patient, Dr. Fitzgerald instructed that an infusion of Haemacell be administered and that the Superintendent prepares and administers the Intravenous cannulation.

I had practised for this moment so simply concentrated on the task in hand – adjust the tourniquet –arm in appropriate position -select the optimum vein- swab the site – uncap the cannula – anchor the vein -smoothly pierce the skin then enter the vein – check blood flash back – slide Teflon cannula fully into the vein – withdraw the steel needle – attach the giving set (already checked for clear flow) to the cannula – start the infusion – check the flow rate and the infusion site for fluid into tissue – all O'K – tape the cannula in place –

Wonderful! my first IV cannulation on scene and I had carried it out well.

QASB CALLS A MEETING RE INFUSION AT SCENE.

Letter from State Council 23.5.84 agreeing to a meeting to discuss Intravenous cannulation by A/Os at scene etc. ref. Dr. Watson

1984 June 28th- full MEETING re A/O'S intravenous cannulation.

Dr. Richard Ashby RBH spoke well, used the tactic that the Casualty Directors Association had looked at PAH and Ipswich for a 'Trial' etc.
Dr. Watson was alert and asked "why?'
Dr. Brophy was negative.
CTO Bob McDermott wants two years for A/Os to be trained in the Training School.
Superintendents Assoc Bob Haswell sees the current trend and supported a "Pilot Scheme." ref. diary notes & letter from Dr. Richard Ashby.

1984 July 19th - second meeting with State Council to discuss a Pilot Scheme for QATB Ipswich.
Drs Brophy, Watson, Fitzgerald, [R. Ashby ill], and Supt. McDonald.
Dr. Brophy was still negative claiming a local anaesthetic injection was required for cannulation - Supt. McDonald remarked that in the 30 years of attending at Casualty departments, he had not witnessed a local anaesthetic being administered to trauma patients for insertion of a cannula for intravenous infusion!
Dr. Watson supportive for Pilot Scheme. ref diary notes

Probably this was the point where the State Council Medical advisers saw that they had lost and Advanced Life Support procedures by qualified Ambulance Officers COULD NOT BE STOPPED so they accepted the face saver of permitting a "Pilot or Trail scheme."

Dr. FitzGerald was now overseas on extended Emergency Department study.

Dr. John Taylor as Director Emergency Department at Ipswich Regional Hospital took up the challenge and was most supportive of ALS by Officers.

CAMPAIGN FOR ALS AT SCENE CONTINUES:

1984 Aug.11- Conference Edwin Tooth Lecture Theatre:
Dr. Harrington re cases in Brisbane take 40 minutes from incident to Hosp.
Dr. Phil Kay speaks on Senior Ambulance Officers infusing, Dr back-up etc
Dr. R. Ashby says Unit with RN's for Cardiac cases not practicable etc.

1984 Aug 30 – discussed the 'letter' from State Council with Dr. Lew Edwards the Deputy Medical Supt. IGH – Dr Edwards supportive of scheme and advised to keep up with Training.
NB: this probably letter stating "A/O's can only infuse with a Doctor present."
Supt. Mc Donald said QATB Ipswich would document all cases which should/could have been infused. examples APPENDIX .

Sept.17 - Dr Noel Stevenson PAH rang and said he had been misquoted, that infusion was still on if 30 minutes or more [away]
Oct. 8 - further discussion re intravenous infusions.

Oct. 29.1984 – only Senior A/Os who have passed theory and practical can carry out intravenous infusion of patients.
Nov.20 – Supt. McDonald successfully administered an intravenous cannulation to a trauma patient at scene. ref: diary entries

Nov. 29.1984 – test for A/O Smith for infusion techniques etc by Dr. Taylor Director Emergency Department at Ipswich Regional Hospital.

The first qualified Officer to request permission to administer intravenous cannulation and infusion to a patient was SAO John Hall.

He was attending an hypoglycaemic patient who had lost consciousness, they were over 30 minutes from Ipswich Hospital.
John radioed Centre control and requested a patch to IGH Emergency Department.

He advised the Medical Officer of the condition of his patient and requested permission to administer an intravenous infusion to reverse the patients condition.

Permission granted and officer Hall finally arrived at Ipswich Hospital with a conscious patient.

CTS – QATB - Central Training School –

March 1985 –F.I.A.O.(Aust.) McDonald gives 'talk' on IAO(Aust.) at QATB Brisbane Centre.
Superintendent Reg Bartels criticises CTO and Training School officers.
He opposes them wanting to expand the CTS whereas he wants an extension to Brisbane Centre. [I didn't agree – CTS must be separate.]

March 29 – McDonald attends Seminar in Adelaide – and 'talks' with South Australia State Ambulance authority officers (ST. John Council).
30-31- March: SA St. John Training Officer criticises Queensland Health Medical Officer on NEC for 'interference' in Training and of being negative.

May 1 – QATB Medical Officer, Dr. Watson rang Supt. Mc Donald to discuss appointment of new Chief Training Officer BUT also discusses Accident Report Form and details of patient Observation as listed.
Supt. McDonald has to inform Dr. Watson that Ipswich A/Os had been using that current Report Form for the past 8 months.

1985 May: – Dr. Phil Kay, Director Emergency Department at Gold Coast Hospital requested Supt. McDonald to present this paper on the "Development of the combined Ambulance/Medical Pre-hospital Care System for Ipswich" to convince Hospital and Ambulance staff of its integrity and success. It was a wet night but a large number of Ipswich staff travelled to support the 'Talk.' copy of Paper available.
This has a good presentation of the different responses of Doctors at an accident scene.

June 4, 1985: Superintend McDonald spoke with State Sec E. Bradley re internal politics with Supt. of Rockhampton the one 'stirring the pot.'
The State Council Secretary admitted that State Council officers were leaking Council business.
Discussed the form of State Ambulance Board and 'the Act'

June 4 - Health Dept : Supt. Invites Dr. Ken Donald Qld. Health Dept. to Presentation night at QATB Ipswich and with other matters speaks about expansion of the Training School and possible changes to the current 'Act.'

Programme next page. ref: Booklet available.

PROGRAMMES

Q.A.T.B. AWARD PRESENTATIONS

INTRODUCTION OF OFFICAL PARTY - M.C. McDONALD, S.B.St.J. F.I.A.O. (AUST) A.A.I.M.

WELCOME OFFICIAL PARTY AND GUESTS - J.J. CUSHING, CHAIRMAN.

ADDRESS BY - DR. KEN DONALD, M.B., B.S., F.R.C.P.A., Ph.D., F.R.A.C.M.A
DEPUTY DIRECTOR GENERAL OF HEALTH AND MEDICAL SERVICES.

PRESENTATION OF CERTIFICATE OF APPRECIATION TO MEDICAL STAFF I.G.H. -

BY DR. KEN DONALD.

RECIPIENT - DR. T. MULHEARN, M.B., B.S., F.R.A.C.S., F.R.C.S.(ED.)
MEDICAL SUPERINTENDENT, IPSWICH GENERAL HOSPITAL.

PRESENTATION OF Q.A.T.B. LONG SERVICE AWARDS - BY DR. KEN DONALD.

RECIPIENTS - SENIOR OFFICER R.H. LATIMORE, 30 YEARS.
STATION OFFICER M.A. SHEPPARD, J.P., 30 YEARS. (RETIRED)
DEPUTY SUPERINTENDENT R. WATSON, 40 YEARS.

PRESENTATION OF NATIONAL MEDALS - BY SIR LLEWELLYN EDWARDS, M.B., B.S., F.R.A.C.M.A

RECIPIENTS - HONORARY OFFICER E.J. CORDINGLEY - NATIONAL MEDAL.
STATION OFFICER O. KNIGHT - NATIONAL MEDAL.
SENIOR OFFICER R.H. LATIMORE - NATIONAL MEDAL & CLASP.
SUPERINTENDENT M.C. McDONALD - CLASP TO NATIONAL MEDAL.
STATION OFFICER J. SMITH - SECOND CLASP TO NATIONAL MEDA

PRESENTATION OF VEHICLE MANOEUVRING (AMBULANCE) - BY J. MARSH, M. Inst. R.S., J.P.
DEPARTMENT OF TRANSPC

RECIPIENTS - AMBULANCE OFFICERS - IPSWICH, BOONAH, GATTON, LAIDLEY, & ROSEWOOD CENTRES.

RESUME - Q.A.T.B. IPSWICH PRE-HOSPITAL CARE SYSTEM - BY J.J. CUSHING, Q.A.T.B. IPSWICH COMMITTEE.

VOTE OF THANKS TO PREVIOUS SPEAKERS - THE HON. W.G. HAYDEN M.P.
MINISTER FOR FOREIGN AFFAIRS.

MR J.J. CUSHING & MEMBERS OF THE COMMITTEE INVITE ALL GUESTS TO LIGHT REFRESHMENTS, & INSPECTION OF PLANS OF Q.A.T.B. IPSWICH CENTRE BUILDINC EXTENSIONS & RENOVATIONS.

June 19 – Supt. McDonald discusses Roles and Objectives and responsibilities of the position etc with future Ipswich Training Officer Neil Kirby and gave same to Officer Kirby for his contemplation – Superintendent to be in control of the Training program etc.

STATE COUNCIL 'AMBULANCE ADMINISTRATION COURSE.'

1985 Aug.29 – Meeting at State Council offices to discuss an 'Ambulance Administration Course.'
Present :- E. Bradley State Council; R. Bartels Superintendents Assoc; M. McDonald, President IAO(Aust.); N. Reece FMWU; D. Brinkhurst TAFE; P. Connelly Exc Health Dept; T. Reader, Chief Training Officer CTS.
The meeting officially formed the "Curriculum Advisory Committee."

NOTE : A.(Tony) READER CHIEF TRAINING OFFICER. diary entry.

1985 Oct 7: Curriculum Advisory Committee framework of Topics.
Nov.21st – draft Course "Ambulance Record Keeping" by M.C. McDonald.
ref. arch file – certificates - records etc. available

STATE COUNCIL MEDICAL ADVISOR TALKS ABOUT PASS/FAIL:-

1985 Nov. 19 – Dr Don Watson rang Supt. McDonald to discuss IV's and entry qualifications so that PASS/FAIL could be introduced etc.
Anyone could call Ipswich Senior Officers 'elite' but this was not the case as the two men worked as a team. Supt. McDonald said Ipswich had the right communications procedures, accreditation to introduce Advanced Care,(or rather acceptable care) etc.
The Superintendent discussed ALS at length and asked that Ipswich be given a Pilot scheme for Defibrillation etc by A/Os now. ref. diary entry

1985 Nov. 27th - letter to QATB from State Council mentions:
(i) " the Redlands experiment, not yet underway"
(ii) the Coronary Unit experiment has Doctors or Nurses present when advanced skills are used –" re Dr. Watson

1985 October – Supt. McDonald as President of the IAO(AUST.) delivered a paper " Medical Teams at the Accident Scene" at the Accident and Emergency Conference at Gold Coast . ref: full Paper available on request
He used this paper to support Ambulance Officers at scene as against Medical Teams attending. The intent was to formally oppose the formation of Hospital Coronary Care Teams which had been proposed.

1985 Dec 12 – Supt. McDonald organised all arrangements and outlined what was required for cardiac monitoring and defibrillation by QATB Ipswich, to Ipswich Hospital Emergency Director Dr. Gerry Fitzgerald and to QASB ATO Kirby – this to be started as a Pilot scheme with Officers John Hall and Anthony Smith.
ref: diary entry.

THE CHANGING OF THE GUARD :

1. 'The Act' is amended and the Queensland Ambulance Service Board is appointed with Gerald Moore Chairman.
2. The composition of the Board does NOT include either a predominance of St. John members nor of Union members, in comparison of the old State Council.
3. 1985 - A. (Tony) Reader is the Central Training School Chief Training Officer.

1986 – May 6 – Superintendent informs Director Emergency Department IGH that Ipswich has all in place for Pre-hospital Coronary Care.

1986 – Oct. Pre hospital Coronary Care Course conducted at QATB Ipswich by Queensland State Council CTS officers and Medicos for 16 Ipswich officers – 14 passed - a 'one of' in Qld. re photo following pages.

1986 July 25 – 7am. Dr Mowatt interim Medical Director Qld. Ambulance appointed by Qld. Health Dept. [not the tame cat a MO wanted] the Doc was very experienced and it was soon obvious he was 'for' the Ambulance officer – he often rang or called on Supt. McDonald.
Dr. Mowatt was a facilitator, adviser, supervisor re Medical regulations etc., later he was an "enforcer" for Coronary Care / Specialists. He was interested in psychology and used this effectively.

12.11.86 Dr. Mowatt requested various Ipswich criteria for appointment and assessment of officers etc.

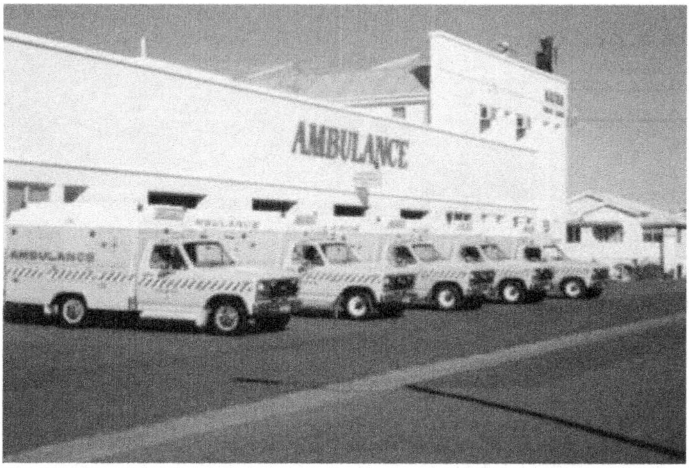

QATB Ipswich Modular Ambulance Units – 1986

Ipswich had introduced a system of replacing the Modular unit on a new F100 chassis every two years as reliable and economic maintenance.

CORONARY CARE INTRODUCED AT QATB IPSWICH:

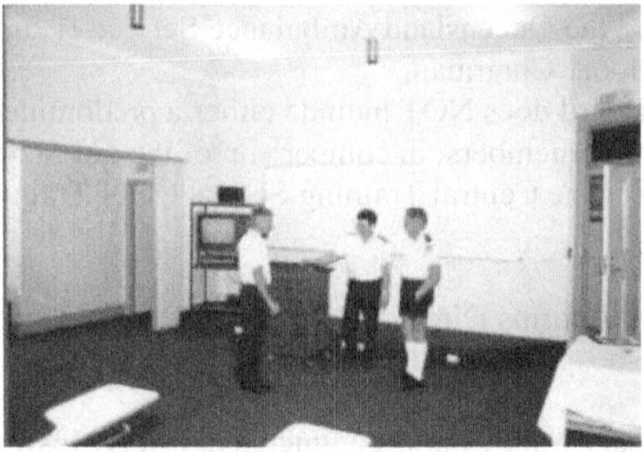

1986 - Office Manager P. Trelour, Supt. McDonald & Station Officer R. Benson check out new Training facility.

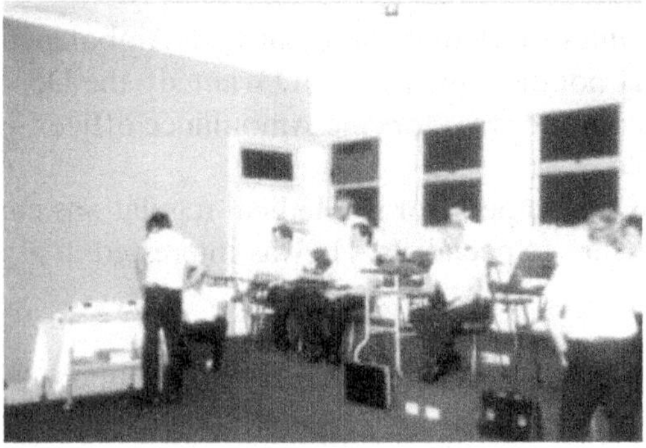

QATB Ipswich Coronary Care officers on Course 1986.

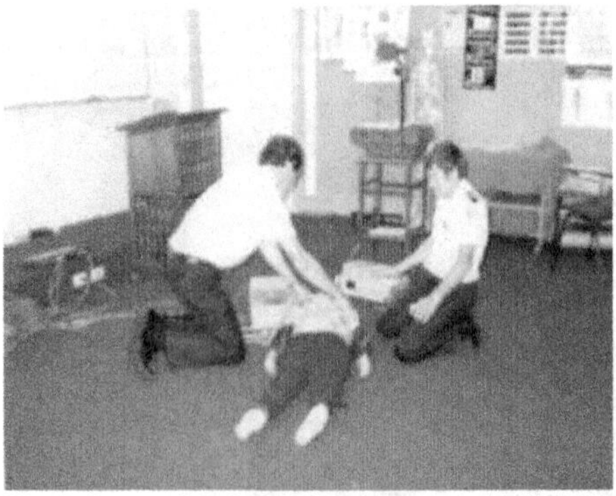

Training with initial Life Pac defibrillator

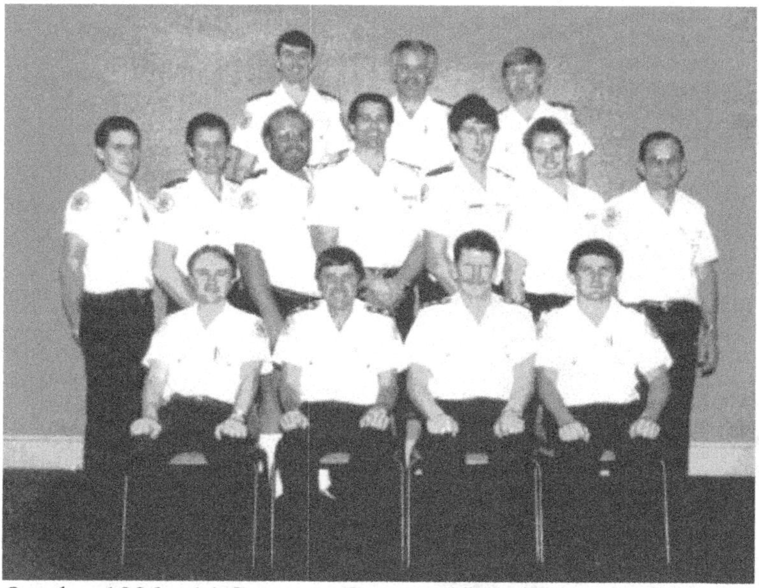

October 1986 – 14 Coronary Care certified officers
A. Smith; J. O'Sullivan; B. Plotski
R. Mc Grigor; R. Henderson; R. Imhoff; J. Hart; S. Picknell; D. Enderman; K. Noie
W. Watson; J. Hall; M. McDonald; J. Strasser

1986 October – 14 Senior Ambulance Officers qualified to administer Pre-hospital Coronary Care – Ipswich now has a Senior Ambulance Officer qualified in Advanced Life Support on each shift– unique for the QATB.

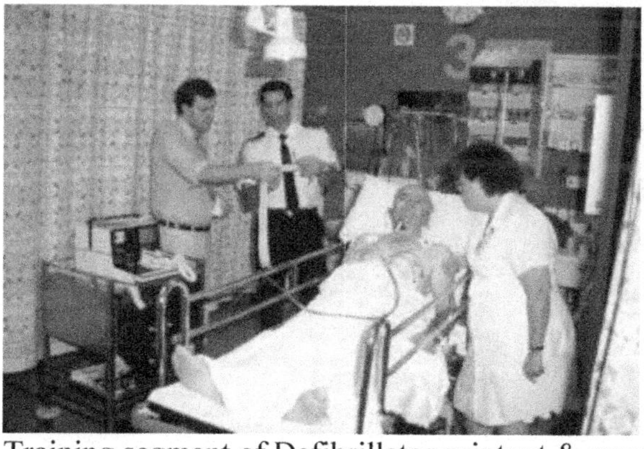

Training segment of Defibrillator printout & report to
Ipswich Hospital Emergency Dept. Dr. FitzGerald;
SAO Hart; ED Charge Sister Brown - new Hewlett-Packard in use.
Ipswich Committee donated their Life Pac defibrillators to IGH.

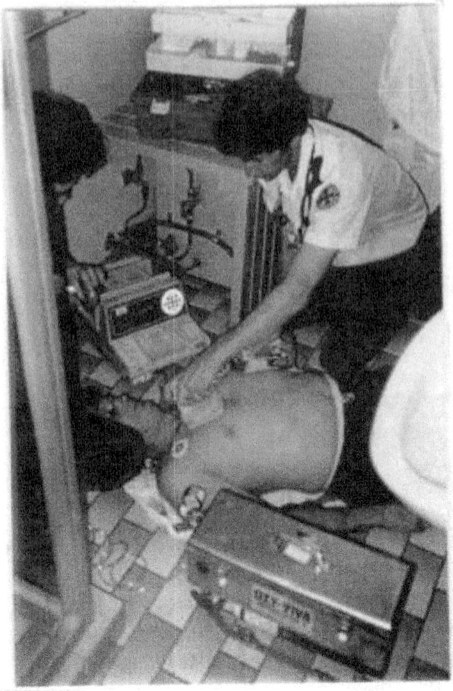

1988 - Training with new Hewlett-Packard Defibrillator
in a confined space scenario
IPSWICH STAFF TRAINING SLIDES FOR SELF STUDY.

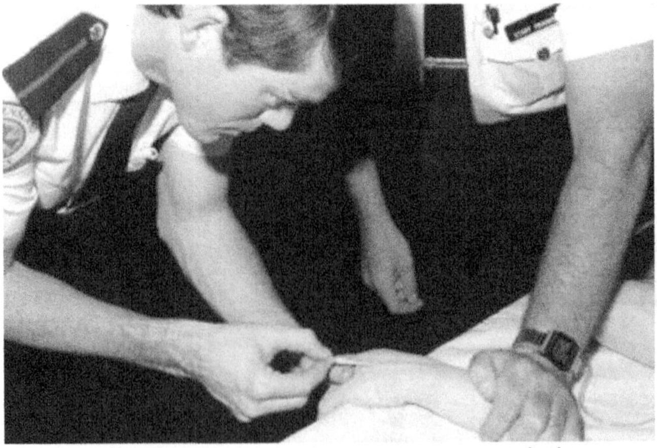

SAO Smith demonstrates intravenous cannulation on a Centre manikin.

A Shot in the Arm.

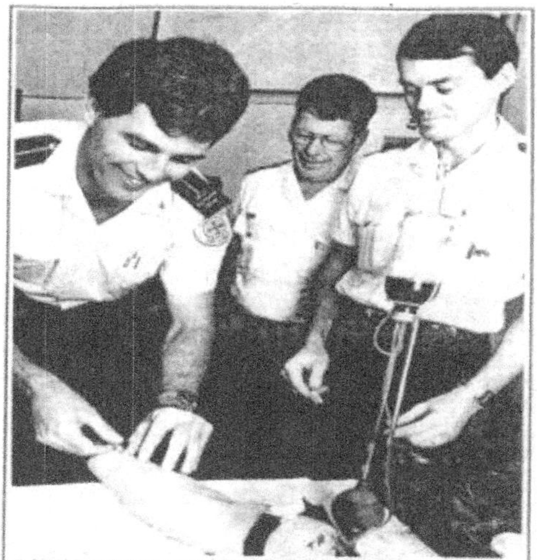

• Ipswich ambulance superintendent Malcolm McDonald (back) watches while skills maintenance officer Daniel Statham (left) and training officer Tony Smith inject their "patient".

SAO Statham the Staff training Maintenance Officer Maintains his cannulation skills and sets up infusion under supervision of SAO Smith and an appreciative Superintendent.

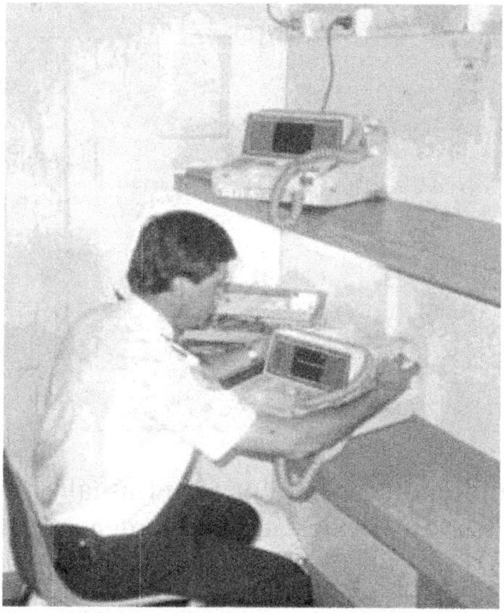

Pre shift check of monitor/defibrillator.

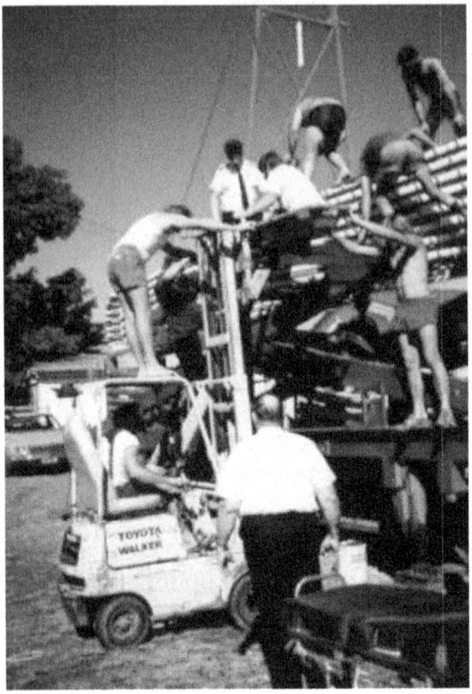

Roof rescue exercise.

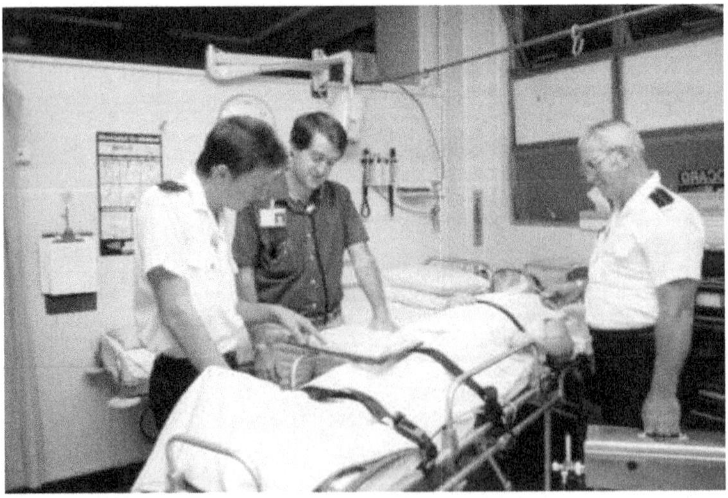

Patient hand-over with Report form to Ipswich Casualty Director Dr. Fitzgerald by Officers R. Bowles and M. Gardener.

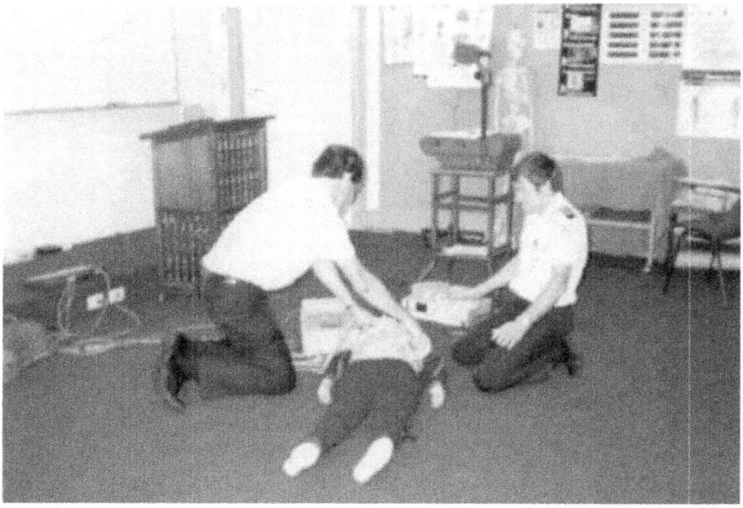

Coronary Care resuscitation exercise – Ipswich Training Room.
Officers J. Hall and D. Statham, using an electronic programmed manikin. Note original Life Pac monitor/defibrillator in the background.

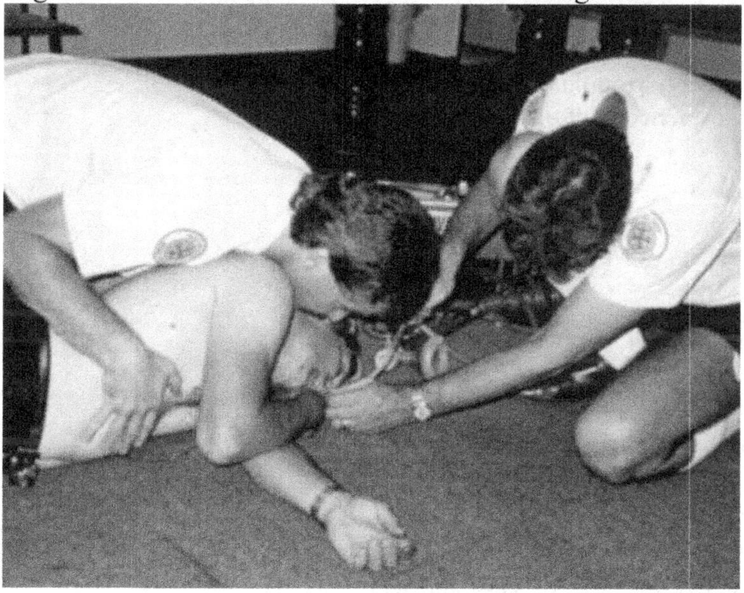

Resuscitation Training 1985 – aspirating patient.

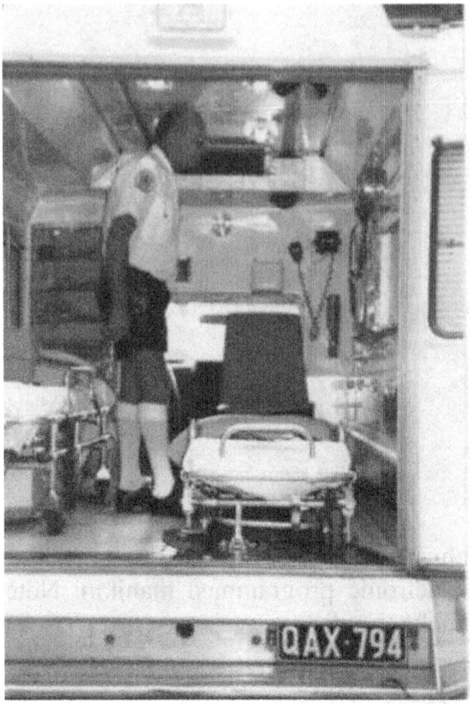

Development of the Ipswich Modular Unit from 1985.
Equipment check at commencement of shift.

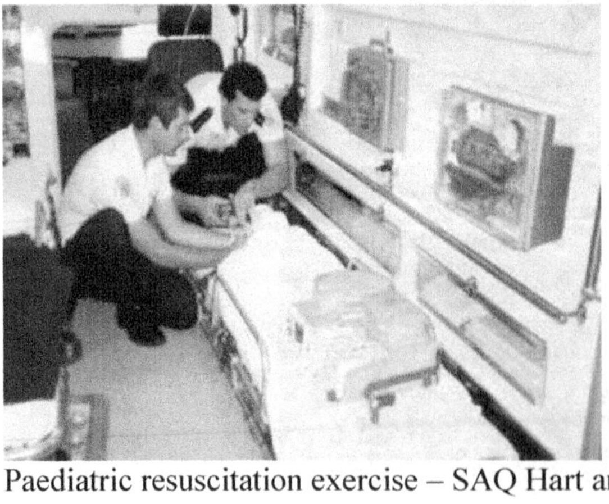

Paediatric resuscitation exercise – SAQ Hart and AO.

ALL IN IT:- the allied services of the Ambulance, Fire and Ipswich Director Emergency Dept. Dr. Taylor attend vehicle accident for Extrication and Emergency care.

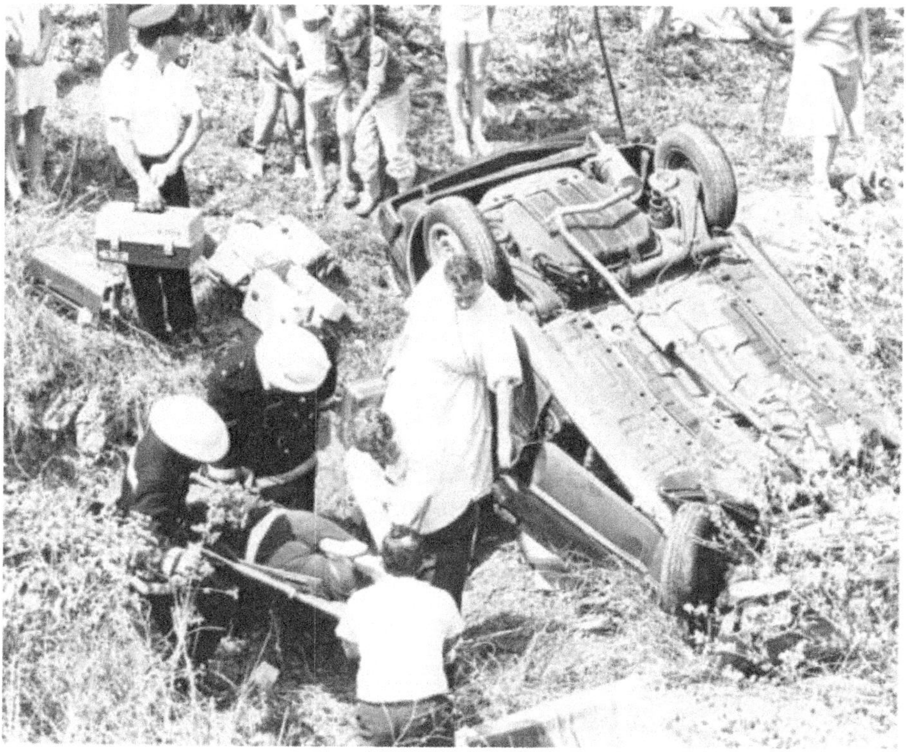

INDUSTRY and PUBLIC FIRST-AID LECTURES.

Superintendent McDonald conducts First-aid classes with allied professional bodies and the respective Staff of local Industry to ensure "the chain of emergency care" is initiated on the shop floor, at local incidents, in the school yard and in the home. This provides the basic climate for successful resuscitation for the intervention of Coronary Care and defibrillation if required.

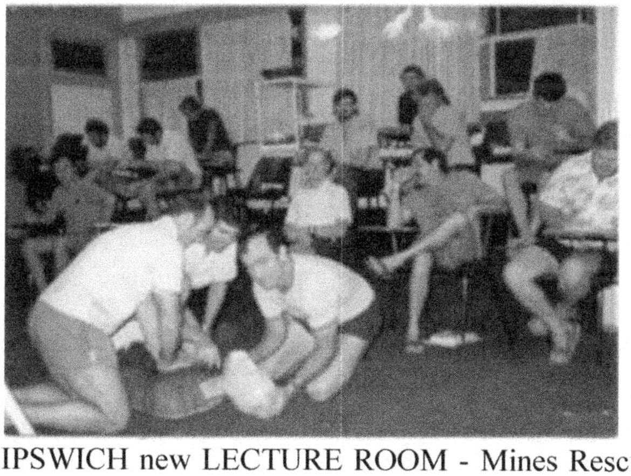

IPSWICH new LECTURE ROOM - Mines Rescue First-aid class, Instructor Supt. McDonald.

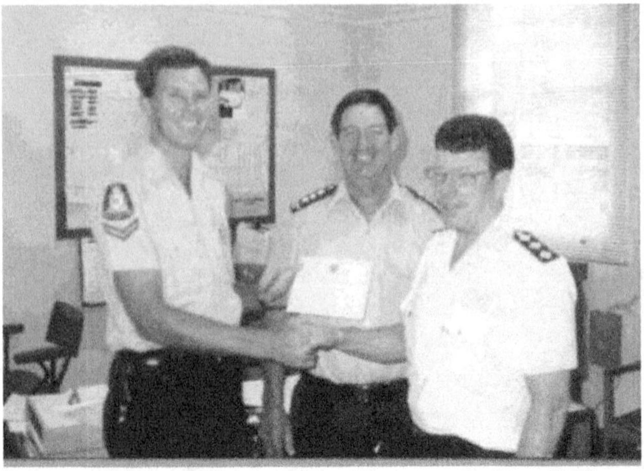

Supt. presents a First-aid certificate to Police Officer.

ANNUAL MEETING OF AUSTRALIAN AMBULANCE AUTHORITIES IN DARWIN, 1986.

1986 Oct. 10th to 19th. Malcolm McDonald, FIAO as President of the IAO(Aust) addressed the combined meeting of Ambulance Authorities in Darwin.

As the first Operational officer to address the AAA he used this opportunity to push the professionalism of Ambulance officers and to pressure the QATB State Council Executive members attending.
This was well received as he was allowed to go well over the time allocated to answer interested questions from the floor.
He continued on the "Qantas Kangaroo tour," meeting with Ambulance executive and Institute members at Alice Springs, Adelaide and Hobart.
He presented a Paper at Adelaide on "Rescue and Retrieval."

Ipswich Centre had reached a level of excellence in the administration of Pre-hospital Emergency Patient care.

1986 December. President McDonald, FIAO, presented a paper on "Rescue and Retrieval" at Surfair Resort Maroochydore.
1986 Dec. 16th. - Officers reassessed (QA) for their Coronary Care qualifications – Supt. McDonald and others passed.

1987 Feb 9 – CTO Bob McDermott rang Superintendent to inform him that Bob was on the Trauma Mortality committee. Superintendent wished him the best but privately feels CTO is 'politically sensitive' with his association with Health.
ref. Diary.

IPSWICH EDUCATION & TRAINING METHODS ADOPTED:

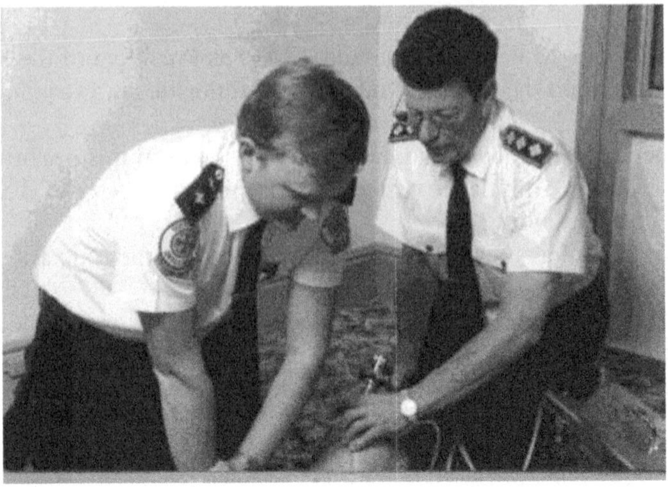

1987- 'Skills maintenance' - Staff Training Officer Kirby and Supt. McDonald.

16.2.87 – QASB suggested Coolangatta learn and use Ipswich Training methods. Nambour requested Ipswich staff entry assessment and criteria.
March 21- Ipswich Training tapes for QATB Cooroy Staff Training in Advanced Life Support. diary
Aug. 11 – QASB Training School advised that the new Medical Director, Dr. Mowatt requested that Ipswich might loan their Training slides of Ipswich Ambulance in action to Dr. Frank Archer in Victoria. Supt. McDonald packed some of his slides and mailed same to Frank. ref. diary
NOTE : The QASB considered QATB Ipswich as delivering Pre-hospital Emergency Care at a standard of excellence and was the example for all Centres to follow.

1987 April 29th - ROLE OF MEDICAL DIRECTOR QASB :
Dr Mowatt rang and discussed concern re rumours – he would have discussed this at length with question and comment, until finally he gave his criteria of the role of the Medical Director :-

- Champion of Ambulance Officer
- Educator
- Loyal to the Health Department.
- Dedicated to the Service.
- Facilitator between Professions.
- Senior Medical Officer (very) to enable discussions with peers, to protect the needs and aspirations of A/O's. diary

I found Dr. Keith Mowatt to be all of these things and gained a respect and friendship for him.

May1st –Superintendent missed reappointment on the Medical Advisory Panel. Doc Mowatt commented that "the M.A.P. was sterile, and there were bigger things for the Superintendent."
E. Bradley had said on 1.4.87 that "McDonald would be looked upon as too close to Metropolitan to be picked for a Representative." diary entry.

Of course this did not reduce my commitment to ensure the patient received 'best practice' at scene with ALS administered by certified Ambulance Officers.

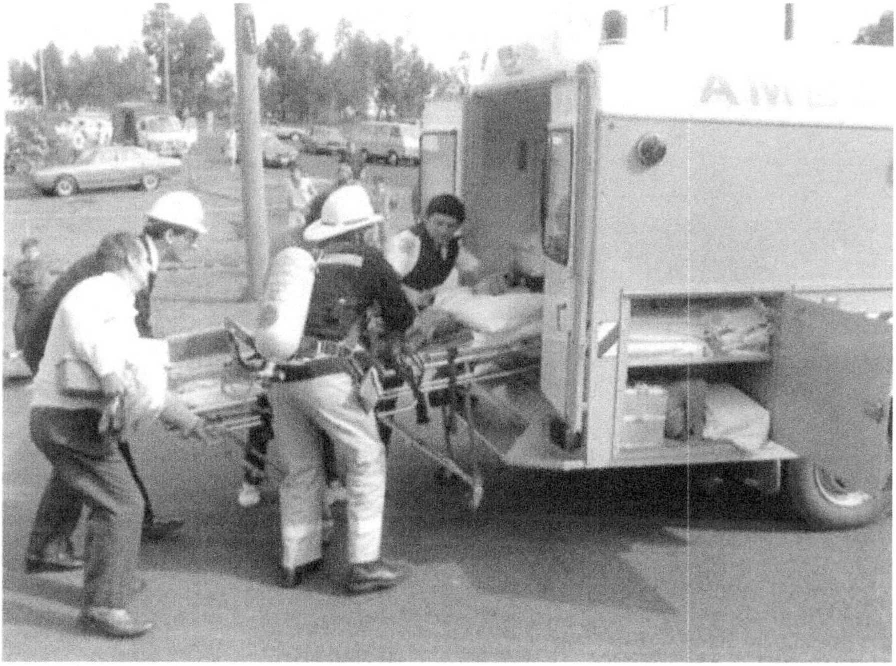

QATB IPSWICH – Rescue of burns victim –TO Kelly and SAO Strasser.

CASE STUDIES and RETROSPECTIVE ANALYSIS.

1987 May - a Reporting program for stats of type, times call out; at scene; left; arr hospital. Whether emergent, resuscitation or injury, was developed and run on the Centre computer using the Call sheets and Accident Report Forms as source core documents – this gave quality control and a visible analysis of results.

Ipswich Computer stats 1987
for analysis of particular category within 24 hours.

Q.A.T.S. (IPSWICH).
CASELOAD x CATEGORY x TIME PERIODS

30-06-87
Page 2

Report for Month of May
for Branch IPSWICH

eg 16 to 6 (morning)

CATEGORY	0-2	2-4	4-6	6-8	8-10	10-12	12-14	14-16	16-18	18-20	20-22	22-24	INVAL	TOTAL
ROAD ACCIDENT														
Cases	4	0	0	3	0	6	2	4	6	1	4	1	0	3[illegible]
Hours	1.72	0.00	0.00	1.99	0.00	1.81	0.15	1.52	3.10	1.00	1.70	0.90	0.00	12.85
Klms	67	0	0	44	0	28	5	18	52	5	17	10	14	260
CHEST PAINS														
Cases	2	1	0	3	3	4	7	5	3	3	2	3	0	36
Hours	1.73	0.78	0.00	2.27	2.87	2.84	4.64	4.07	3.02	2.59	1.13	2.99	0.00	26.9[illegible]
Klms	15	16	0	25	32	37	46	61	80	31	17	51	0	419
URGENT MEDICAL														
Cases	3	3	1	9	21	15	14	12	8	8	8	10	0	112
Hours	2.72	2.65	0.85	7.02	14.74	10.35	6.62	8.67	6.87	6.87	5.24	6.27	0.00	80.67
Klms	47	47	11	138	219	173	227	98	184	145	76	133	0	1496
OTHER														
Cases	0	0	0	8	19	21	8	21	21	6	8	6	7	125
Hours	0.00	0.00	0.00	20.96	42.34	52.28	4.73	13.94	3.41	1.83	26.93	2.17	0.00	168.5[illegible]
Klms	0	0	0	101	154	166	77	177	72	23	62	54	52	938
RESUSITATION														
Cases	0	0	0	0	1	0	0	0	0	0	0	0	0	1
Hours	0.00	0.00	0.00	0.00	0.73	0.00	0.00	0.00	0.00	0.00	0.00	0.00	0.00	0.73
Klms	0	0	0	0	8	0	0	0	0	0	0	0	0	8
URGENT SURGICAL														
Cases	0	0	0	1	0	1	0	0	0	0	0	0	0	2
Hours	0.00	0.00	0.00	0.72	0.00	0.35	0.00	0.00	0.00	0.00	0.00	0.00	0.00	1.07
Klms	0	0	0	7	0	8	0	0	0	0	0	0	0	15
TRAUMA														
Cases	4	0	1	4	6	5	10	15	10	6	3	3	0	57
Hours	2.61	0.00	1.13	2.01	3.00	4.25	5.69	12.00	8.17	4.67	0.97	2.88	0.00	47.36
Klms	37	0	23	35	38	75	102	241	174	105	16	39	26	911
WHITE														
Cases	6	3	5	319	269	318	273	201	62	23	24	10	18	[illegible]
Hours	5.62	3.15	2.27	277.90	115.98	145.29	158.31	104.41	40.92	16.30	19.04	5.21	0.00	894.4[illegible]
Klms	199	93	70	3644	2803	3405	3789	2516	966	335	500	125	334	[illegible]
TOTAL CASES	13	7	7	347	319	370	314	250	130	47	49	33	25	[illegible]
TOTAL HRS.	14.40	6.58	4.85	312.87	179.66	217.17	182.14	144.61	65.49	33.26	55.0[illegible]	20.42	0.00	1235.86
TOTAL KLMS	365	156	112	3994	3254	3892	4246	3113	1550	704	688	412	425	22927

1987 Nov.10 – Dr Mowatt spoke to Supt. McDonald re 'Blueprint for Ambulance in Queensland.'

- base line>
- implementation >
- supportive action >
- raise standards >
- action to be taken.

Medical Director requested :- Since Ipswich has worked toward Certification and the implementation of intravenous infusion at scene etc and suffered investigation, and had successfully defended the action.

That Ipswich to set qualifications and allow Ambulance Officer from Emerald to carry out intravenous cannulation training with support from Central Training School etc and that Resource Officer Fred Marnock to work for one day at Ipswich.

	1987		1988		1989		1990	
Total Arrests	54		57		80		68	
Defibrillated	33	61.30%	28	49.20%	41	52.00%	34	50.00%
Saves	6	18.00%	4	14.20%	4	9.90%	5	14.70%
Witnessed Arrests	1	1.850%	10	17.50%	9	11.40%	3	4.480%
Males	43	80.00%	34	65.00%	53	67.00%	50	74.00%
Females	11	20.00%	20	35.00%	26	33.00%	18	26.00%
Location of Arrests	47	Homes	43	Homes	63	Homes	54	Homes
	2	Dr's Surg	1	Dr's Surg			2	Dr's Surg
	2	Sporting			1	Sporting	1	Sporting
	1	Shopping	1	Shopping	5	Shopping	3	Shopping
	1	Work					1	Work
	1	Road	1	Road	2	Road	2	Road
			1	Hospital	1	Hospital		
			2	Rail Stn	2	Rail Stn		
			1	Church	1	Church		
			6	Ambulance				
			1	Police Stn				
					1	Social	1	Hotel
					1	School	1	School

		1987	1988	1989	1990
Total Arrests		54	57	80	68
Defibrillated		33 or 61.3%	28 or 49.2%	41 or 52.0%	34 or 50.0%
Saves		6 or 18.0%	4 or 14.2%	4 or 9.9%	5 or 14.7%
Witnessed Arrests		1 or 1.85%	10 or 17.5%	9 or 11.4%	3 or 4.48%
Sex Ratio	Males	43 or 80.0%	34 or 65.0%	53 or 67.0%	50 or 74.0%
	Females	11 or 20.0%	20 or 35.0%	26 or 33.0%	18 or 26.0%

Average response times to all = 5.4 minutes / Average response to *saves* only = 3.9 minutes

STATISTICAL DATA ON CORONARY CARE
OVER FOUR CALENDER YEARS, 1987, 1988, 1989, 1990

NOTE: 'SAVES' walked away from Hospital on discharge.

DISASTER EXERCISE MINDEN RANGE – QATB IPSWICH. 15.9.1987

Mock rescue near Minden

By SARA HEATON

MORE than 100 emergency services workers took part in a dramatic mock rescue exercise on the Minden Range on Tuesday night.

The disaster was modelled on the crash at Cairns early this year when a bus plunged over a mountain side, killing eight students and injuring 32 others, plus the bus driver and two teachers.

Police, ambulance, fire brigade, hospital, 70 State Emergency Service personnel and the Salvation Army worked together to test their skills and equipment in coping with a major disaster.

Venturer Scouts from the Moreton Division acted out the roles of the dead and injured from a bus and car crash during the two-hour exercise, which began at 7pm.

A committee of eight emergency service workers acted as observers to assess the exercise.

A debriefing meeting will be held next Thursday to discuss any problems observed.

Esk council graded a ramp where a bus donated by Minden Bus Service was parked to simulate a crash at the bottom of a hill.

Workers had to remove passengers trapped in a wrecked car and transport injured up a steep 100m incline.

Ten were dead, 10 seriously injured and 20 injured, but mobile. Each person carried a list of injuries and were briefed on their nature so they could answer questions from ambulance workers.

Doctors and nursing staff from Ipswich Hospital Accident and Emergency department and a medical resuscitation team were involved in the exercise.

Ambulance co-ordinator and Ipswich Superintendant Malcolm McDonald said the exercise overall was successful.

Supt McDonald was pleased with the way staff coped with problems presented by the site of the accident and the congestion at the top of the hill.

Harborview Medical Center

325 NINTH AVENUE
SEATTLE, WASHINGTON 98104
206 223-3000

May 16, 1988

Mr. Malcolm C. McDonald, A.I.A.O, (Australia)
Superintendent
Ipswich Center
Queensland Ambulance Transport Brigade
P.O. Box 408
Ipswich, Queensland 4305 AUSTRALIA

Dear Superintendent McDonald;

I enjoyed every minute of your seemingly innocent, but very carefully arranged, Ipswich Coronary Care and Pre-Hospital Life Support Seminar.

Not only was I able to watch a man with impeccable political credentials at work, but I also had fun. I credit you with putting my wife in the position of having to refuse a last banana-sized shrimp. That privilege I do not take lightly.

I appreciate the graciousness of your introductions during the conference, and for opening your home to provide the best luncheon we experienced in Australia.

I hope that you continue to enjoy driving the State of Queensland in the direction of progress. Thank you again for your courtesy and most generous hospitality.

Respectfully,

Michael K Copass

Michael K. Copass, M.D.
Professor of Medicine/Neurology

Medical Director
Emergency Trauma Center
Harborview Medical Center

Deputy Director, Director of Training
Seattle Medic One

MKCjsm

a component of the Warren G. Magnuson Health Sciences Center of the University of Washington

PASS/FAIL CERTIFICATION :

1988 Aug. 30. Dr. Mowatt conferred with Supt. McDonald re 'where are we going' and PASS/FAIL – McDonald says PASS/FAIL for all courses NOW.
Dr. Mowatt rang back. He had discussed this with the QASB Administrator Ian Boddice that the service had to be professional, had to have pass/fail throughout, and a criteria for entry?
Ian Boddice gave the task to the Medical Director to 'work it out.' Diary.

DEVET and **Ambulance Administration Course subjects**.
1989 April 6 & May – DEVET McDonald invited onto Course Assessment Committee regarding Toowoomba College and Ambulance Administration subjects. Ref. Arch file certs/records/etc

1990 March 14 – Minister for Health consulted with Supt. McDonald regarding Ambulance coming back to Health [there was pressure for Health to retain Ambulance service] McDonald replied that the QATB needed finance to progress and QATB wanted its identity in relation to Pre-hospital Emergency Patient Care protected not lost. diary entry

1990 May 1st – Major William Sng National University Hospital of Singapore – out to study Ambulance service – QASB sent him to Supt. McDonald at Ipswich for his full period in Australia.

Major William Sng National University Hospital Singapore , studies Ipswich Ambulance Service System. May 1990

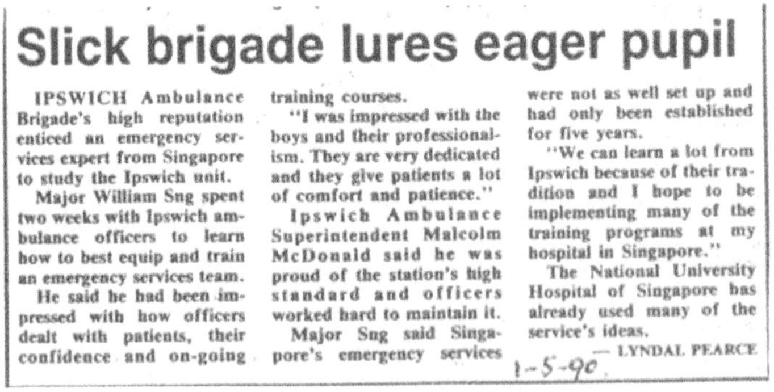

Slick brigade lures eager pupil

IPSWICH Ambulance Brigade's high reputation enticed an emergency services expert from Singapore to study the Ipswich unit.

Major William Sng spent two weeks with Ipswich ambulance officers to learn how to best equip and train an emergency services team.

He said he had been impressed with how officers dealt with patients, their confidence and on-going training courses.

"I was impressed with the boys and their professionalism. They are very dedicated and they give patients a lot of comfort and patience."

Ipswich Ambulance Superintendent Malcolm McDonald said he was proud of the station's high standard and officers worked hard to maintain it.

Major Sng said Singapore's emergency services were not as well set up and had only been established for five years.

"We can learn a lot from Ipswich because of their tradition and I hope to be implementing many of the training programs at my hospital in Singapore."

The National University Hospital of Singapore has already used many of the service's ideas.

— LYNDAL PEARCE

1-5-90.

OPERATION " SILICIA" May 1990.

1990 May 17 – Operation " Silica" Ipswich carries the major role for the firm and assists with at scene Advanced Life Support procedures. To test the 'Emergency Procedure' of the James Hardie factory in Carole Park – both organisations benefitted. ref: Press report & photos.

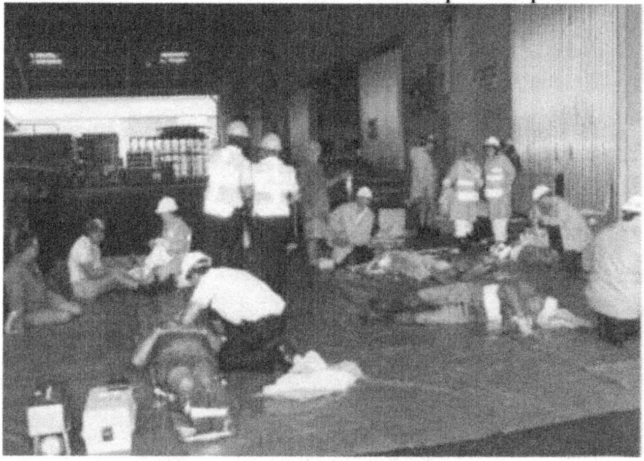

Operation 'Silica' Dr. T. Choong, Casualty Director in red helmet; Ambulance Casualty Officers, SAOs Leader and Plotski in yellow helmets.

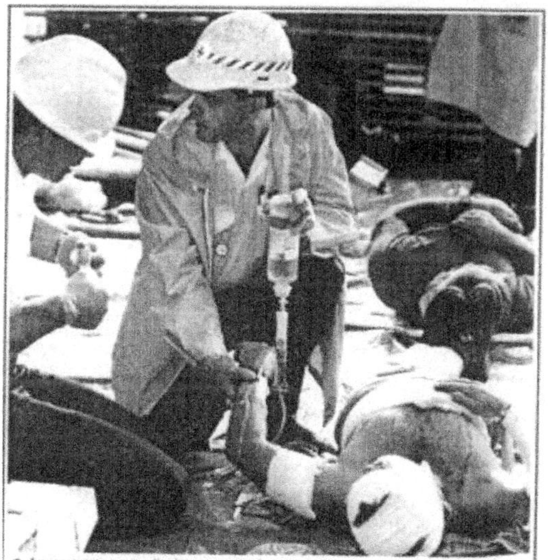

• An emergency medical team puts in some practice yesterday at the James Hardie factory in Carole Park.

Operation "Silica" 17.5.1990 a Major Incident exercise. Ipswich qualified Sen. Ambulance Officers cannulate a patient at scene and set up for an infusion in the 'Casualty Clearing Station.'

1990 June – Press Report, "an emergency technique initiated by Ipswich Ambulance about seven years ago is being trailed across Queensland for introduction throughout the State." Qld. Times Press cutting -attached

/ 805

READY ALWAYS

QUEENSLAND AMBULANCE TRANSPORT BRIGADE

IPSWICH COMMITTEE

Your Ref

19th April, 1990 Our Ref MCMcD:lw

Mr I. Boddice,
Manager,
Q.A.S.B.,
P.O. Box 251.
SOUTH BRISBANE. 4101

Dear Sir,

RE: EXERCISE 'SILICA' 17TH MAY, 1990

As you are aware, exercise 'Silica' is a major multi-casualty accident exercise to be conducted at the James Hardie Wacol Factory on Thursday 17th May, 1990, at 1000 hours.

The above exercise is under the organisation of the Police Operational Planning Unit Brisbane.

A number of meetings have been held under the Chairmanship of Inspector Norm Sprenger who is also responsible for the dissemination of all minutes and instructions relating to the exercise.

From these meetings, certain people have been alloted specific tasks, one of which is the situation arrangements, casualty list, injuries and exercise organisation. Training Officer Kelly, Doctor Mark Waters, Mary Reid and Studio One have met at various times and have this well in hand.

It is recognised that as the multi-casualty incident will originate at James Hardie and Company Wacol Factory within the Ipswich area, then the Q.A.T.B. Ipswich multi-casualty plan will be initiated after a call for assistance is received at the Q.A.T.B. Ipswich Centre.

Objective 5.3 is to practice the response and co-ordination of Ambulance and other authorities, therefore Ipswich will be incorporating the sections of our Plan which require assistance from neighbouring Centres. To this end Ipswich has invited participation from Brisbane, Beenleigh and Zone Centres.

Q.A.T.B. Ipswich will be organising a 'briefing' with Ambulance Centres on the Ambulance involvement in this exercise, prior to 'the day'.

Yours faithfully,

M.C. McDonald

M.C. McDONALD,
Superintendent & Secretary.

Cnr. Downs & Flint Sts., NORTH IPSWICH 4305
All Communications to be addressed to the Secretary — P.O. Box 408, IPSWICH 4305
Telephones: Emergency: 000. Transports: (07) 281 1000.

COLLISION WARREGO HIGHWAY.

Two vehicle collision Warrigo Highway plus one:

The call came in: 'two vehicles have collided on the Warrigo highway, a car and a truck"
QATB Ipswich Control despatched one Emergency Unit immediately and diverted a second unit from a routine case to back-up.

On arrival SO Smith reported, " on scene, one patient, conscious, from a car which overturned off the highway, a second patient, unconscious, is trapped in another car which is heavily damaged from impact with a semitrailer, will require Medical assistance, secondary report will follow."

The Control Officer followed the Emergency Procedure for entrapment and informed the Superintendent, of the situation and the request for Medical assistance.

I immediately ceased what I was doing and hurried to the retrieval Unit and preceded to the Ipswich Hospital to collect the Medical Officer being arranged by Control with Dr. Thomas Choong the Director of Emergency Department.

I collected the MO and proceeded to the crash site with all possible speed, as 20 minutes would have already elapsed from the time of impact.

Siren off - there was the crash scene before us - a major highway - cars and trucks backed up for a kilometre - red and blue lights flashing from Police, Ambulance and Fire units - further units arriving on scene to assist in the extrication and treatment of the casualties, and to bring the chaotic congestion under control.

On our arrival my role was Scene Commander/ Ambulance > out of the unit > eyes sweeping the scene > crumpled mass of a car impacted on the front of a semitrailer > an overturned car just off the road > officer was moving a patient from that vehicle to one of the Ambulance units.

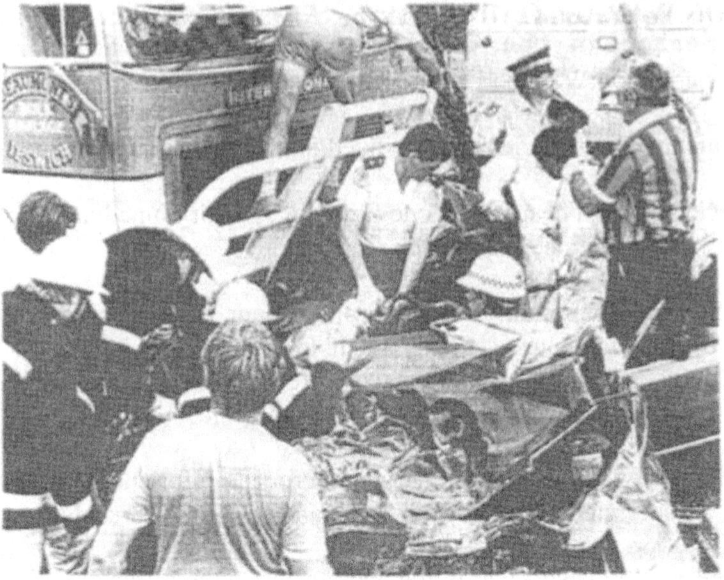

THE SCENE

THE SMELL - of engine exhausts - hot engines - burnt rubber from sudden and vicious braking.

THE NOISE - NOISE EVERYWHERE - motors of Fire, Police and Ambulance units running, (they must charge the batteries for lights, 2 way radio, equipment), - the sharper engine note of the power generator for the hydraulic rescue cutters and spreaders - the deep diesel roar of the mobile crane which had been commandeered by the Police Co-ordinator.

At scene are three Ambulance units and crews, one Fire tender and a Rescue Appliance, with four Police units with officers to Co-ordinate and facilitate all requirements for the Emergency services at scene and to control the traffic congestion on the Highway and to protect the Emergency personal at scene.

On our arrival Senior A/O Smith stepped away from the wreckage to provide myself and the Medical Officer with a Situation Report - the casualty from the second car had received Primary Care, was not seriously injured and had been loaded into one Unit - the male person in the wreckage was unconscious with multiple injuries. The driver of the Semi was unhurt and under observation.

As I stepped towards the trapped patient I indicated that the loaded Ambulance Unit proceed to Ipswich hospital immediately - the MO checked the trapped patient.

The extensive damage to the car made it very difficult for the Ambulance officers to fully assess and to treat the patient.

Officers Smith and Bain had to work through the damaged passenger's door in a very restricted area.

The patient was unconscious – bleeding from the mouth and nose .

He was surrounded by twisted metal making it very difficult to maintain an open airway – suction was used – the patient was being ventilated with 100% oxygen by bag and mask – blood had to be wiped from his face and the mask repeatedly.
The Senior Fire Officer informed me that they were in the process of removing the hood from the car to allow access for our officers.

I observed the shocked condition of the patient, his slumped posture, and the wreckage from a high velocity impact – I indicated the airway management and ventilation continue.
I directed neck support to be applied, and tasked a junior officer with supplying necessary equipment from Units nearby, and to maintain a check on all equipment.

The Medical Officer decided to cannulate the patient via his left arm which he could just reach between the damaged seats, Senior Officer Smith assisted.

The Fire team had cut through the hood supports and now removed the hood off the damaged car.
This gave the Medical and Ambulance Officers better access to the patient albeit still with some difficulty.

I directed Training Officer Kelly to prepare for infusion by way of veins in the patients right arm in case this was needed due to his multiple injuries and blood loss.
The Medical Officer reassessed the patient as having head and facial injuries, injury to his lower limbs which were still trapped in the twisted metal of what had once been a car.
I asked him if he required further assistance, and might I have the Emergency Director attend?
I requested the Police Co-ordinator to contact IGH and have the Director of Emergency Department transported to the scene.

The patient was still trapped by his lower limbs but now that the hood had been removed, a cervical stiff neck collar had been applied, he was receiving assisted ventilation with 100% oxygen, his airway maintained by an artificial airway and aspiration – secondary assessment and vital signs recorded, intravenous infusion running via veins in this left arm.

Fire officers used hydraulic jaws to push the twisted body metal apart, working to free his lower limbs.
The Police Co-ordinator asked if I wanted the crane to lift part of the car wreckage to help free the patient – "YES."
CREAK! SOME MOVEMENT OF TWISTED METAL –"NO! – HOLD IT"

Dr. Thomas Choong arrived, I gave him a full update, he decided to intubate the patient due to his condition and the difficulty in maintaining a clear airway and for manual ventilation of the patient.

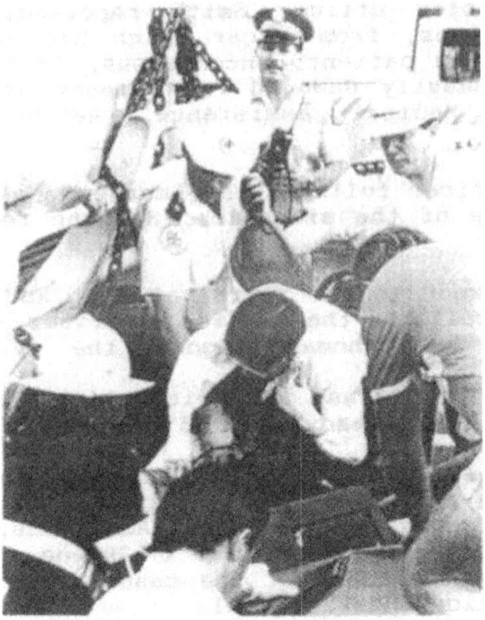

Dr. Choong on scene examining trapped patient – Police Co-ordinator background.
Red safety helmet 'a must' for the Doctor.

The patient's foot was freed which allowed his extrication from the wreck, so intubation was delayed until he was loaded into the Ambulance.

With great care the patient was lifted from the wreck – there was no limit to assistants from Fire and Police officers working with A/Os – all following my direction as a team to ensure all injuries were supported and his airway maintained - like a many armed caterpillar – a bystander holding the 'intravenous drip' elevated. He was then lowered onto the stretcher and transferred into the Ambulance.

Whilst DR. Choong intubated the patient with the assistance from the MO and SAO Smith, thus ensuring an open and protected airway, other Ambulance Officers applied a Thomas splint to align and stabilise the fractured femur and a splint to the fractured arm, etc.

I requested a Police escort for the Ambulance to provide a steady uninterrupted transport to Ipswich hospital, and to clear the route through the traffic congestion.

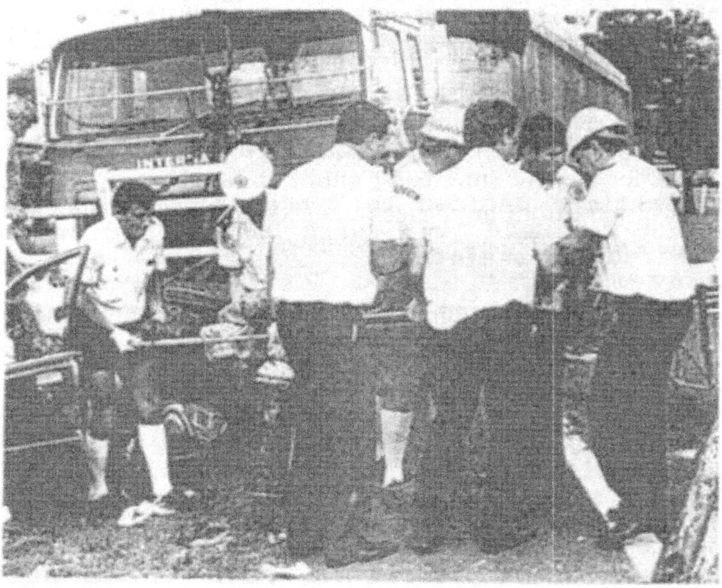

Extrication effected and transferred into the Ambulance.
A full team effort of Medical, Ambulance, Police and Fire Services.

Some months later a letter of Commendation from R. Dargusch, Assistant Commissioner, Police Southern Region was received by Deputy Superintendent John Hall on the excellent work performed at scene on 19 October 1990 and naming all Officers involved on the case for their professionalism and dedication to duty.
ref: appendix

It was most appreciated coming from an allied Service who was just as involved.

NOTE: by this time the QATB Central Training School had taken from IPSWICH :-
Chief Training Officer; Tony Reader.
Training Officer: Neil Kirby.
Training Officer: Martin Kelly
Resource Officer: Mark McDonald.

1990 - Supt. McDonald submits letters to Minister and to the Director General with discussion on some proposed changes to the structure of the QATB.

SORRY, WE CAN'T GO: trapped patient emergency.

Val had been to the hairdresser earlier in the day, and had then prepared for us to attend the Rotary function that night.

I'd finished work for the day, informed Control of my plans and walked home, that is, I walked downstairs from my office, along the footpath to the other end of the Centre building then up the stairs to our residence.

A leisurely bath and dressed for an expected enjoyable dinner and night at Rotary, put on the best 'mocka' and we were ready to leave by about six-thirty.

I had heard an Ambulance unit depart earlier, so when the phone rang I assumed Control was going to inform me of the situation before I left - foolish fellow that I was.

I picked up the handset," Super here," I answered.

"Super, we've got an emergency of a man trapped under a truck, and the Officer has requested Medical back-up and Rescue, says we might need a crane," came the statement from Control.

The Procedures I had in place listed that the Superintendent be informed of any emergency requiring Medical back-up or entrapment, allowing the Superintendent to direct further action.

" Right I'll be over, ring the Hospital and arrange for me to pick up a senior Casualty Department Medico, notify the Police, and the Fire Brigade, alert another crew to standby," I instructed according to our Procedures.

I hurried into our lounge room where Val was waiting, she glanced at me and a look of resignation showed on her face before I spoke, **" SORRY LOVE WE CAN'T GO,** a man's trapped, doesn't sound too good, might be a while," I said as I pulled off my tie and continued out the door.

The Retrieval station sedan was ready for me when I walked into the Centre, and I drove off to the hospital. I checked radio reception with Control and received directions and an update on the situation.
The Assistant Director of Casualty, Dr John Taylor was waiting for me at the hospital so no time was lost, and we arrived at scene in about ten minutes.

As in most cases the message received does not always give the full story, but now in front of us, in the light of the cars headlights was the true picture.
In front of us was an overturned semi-trailer, but the driver's cabin of the semi was smashed flat by an 11 tonne tractor, WHICH WAS STILL **ON TOP OF THE**

CABIN, and the driver was **STILL IN THE CABIN**, what hope ?

I picked up my portable radio and John and I stepped out of the car and hurried over to the senior Ambulance officer,
" What's the situation Bob ?" I asked, as I looked at the wreckage, and the large, heavy tractor balanced above.

" Well Super," he replied," we're really not sure how the bloke is, only to say he could be alive, cause at this stage we can only just see one foot."

Looking at the wreckage we wondered if that really meant anything.

I now became aware that I was standing in soft clay soil in good shoes, in good clothes, and wearing rose gold cuff links handed down from my Father, in my shirt sleeves.

Oh well, that's part of the job, I mused as I removed my treasured cuff links and secured them in my fob pocket.

Police and Fire officers arrived and we three Commanders discussed the situation.

Debris had to be carefully removed to gain some access to the patient, to allow assessment of his condition and to provide whatever emergency treatment he required to the limits of our access.

Secondly the tractor was about 11 tonne, sitting on top of the crushed cabin and the driver, and above any rescuers, so it's removal had to be under strict supervision to avoid further injury to the driver, and any injury to us.

The Police Scene Commander decided to requisition a heavy crane, the crane had to lift 11 tonne, and the Fire Scene Commander would supervise gaining entry to the patient if safety allowed.

After some careful digging under the crushed metal we could see down this gap about a four inch area of the patient's face.

Shortly the driver answered our repeated question of, " are you alright mate," to check if he was conscious, by a croaked, " yeh " - you beaut, he's alive and now conscious.
To further questions, he could only say that he could not move, and did not have much feeling due to the pressure of the wreckage.
We hoped that the weight was the only problem he had, but if this was sustained then there was real danger from soft tissue trauma also.

I examined the other side of the crushed cabin and found a small gap which might allow one of my slightly built officers to just reach out and touch the driver.

I instructed Officer Grant Gamble on what I wanted, for him to try and reach the patient, to ascertain his skin temperature - whether hot or cold, also if the skin was moist or dry.

Grant squirmed into the gap and strained to reach the patient until he was successful, and was able to report that the patient's skin appeared normal.

Good, I ordered him out and informed Dr. Taylor and Dr. Fitzgerald of the examination.

The situation had attracted Media attention, which had brought a concerned inquiry from the Minister for Health, Hon. William Knox, and an offer of helicopter assistance from the Royal Brisbane Hospital, but we had the situation under control.

The crane arrived and manoeuvred into position, with a professional 'dogman' riding the hook.

Heavy chains were attached to the tractor chassis, and tension taken on the crane cable in response to the Dogman's whistled instructions.

AO Imhoff and I spoke to the driver, informing him of all that was happening, and I had one hand on a protruding piece of wreckage to gauge if it shifted when the crane lifted the tractor.

A sharp blast on the Dogman's whistle - the crane cable tightened - two sharp blasts - THE TRACTOR TWISTED - the crane stopped - it's too dangerous.

By this time a crowd of better than one hundred people had gathered and numbers were still growing, the Police have ordered them onto the slope behind the scene, away from the water table.

Regroup of Scene Commanders and the Crane operator, it is decided to adjust the chains and try again.

Whistle from the Dogman - lift of the crane cable - shift of the tractor - STOP.

It is then decided to wait for two bulldozers, and to position them with their blades steadying the tractor, the crane to lift, and the dozers to push and swing the tractor off to one side.

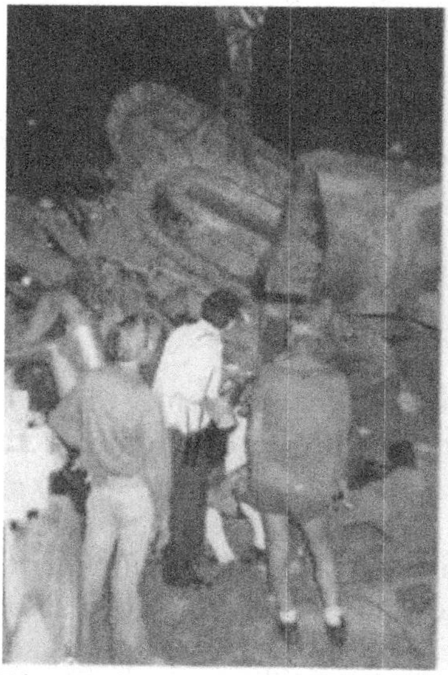
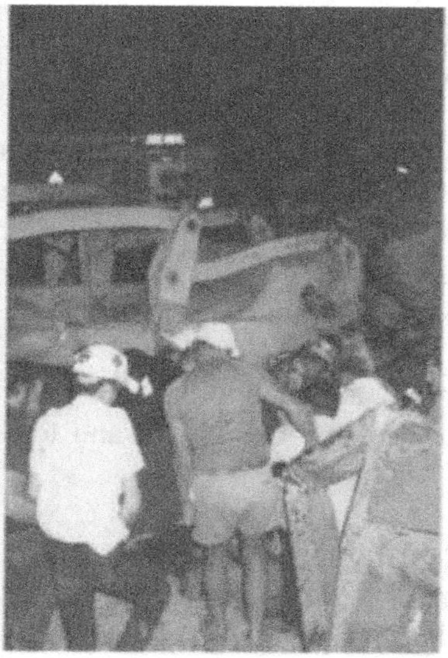

The 11 tonne Tractor is balanced, it is a dangerous position.

The injured driver is 'stretchered' out.

Bob and I were beside the wreck, Bob talking to the driver and I was there to direct and on guard to warn Bob and pull him out of the way,[I hoped], if the tractor started to slide our way.

A blast from the Dogman - roar of power from the two dozers - the crane cable tightens - the blades of the dozers are against the tractor - THE TRACTOR TWISTS - the Dogman signals - the dozers roar and push - the tractor is clear - the dozers push forward - all's over - the tractor is on the ground - a ROAR from the crowd.

Willing hands jacked up the wrecked cabin with hydraulic spreaders, and we carefully lifted the driver out and onto a stretcher, then into the Ambulance unit to examine him fully.

Incredible, he had suffered a fractured wrist, some small lacerations, a lot of bruising, but no major injuries.

We splinted his arm, treated his wounds, put up a drip for drug therapy and in case of internal injury, and drove off after two and a half hours.

It was a dangerous situation, where people could have been injured, and the patient and/or ambulance personnel could have lost their lives, but all parties acted professionally, respecting each other's role, and the job was managed with deliberation and expertise.
A great team effort, but a typical situation met by Ambulance officers in their daily duties.

THE 1990 SELECT COMMITTEE OF INQUIRY INTO AMBULANCE SERVICES

The 1990 Select Committee of Inquiry into Ambulance Services was a bi-patrician Parliamentary Committee of Inquiry with the voting power in the control of the Government of the day, BUT, it was the umpteenth Inquiry into the Ambulance Service and one wondered if this would actually introduce needed changes or simply put the findings into the 'too hard basket' just as previous Inquiries had done.

Members of the Committee attended at Ipswich Centre to interview people who had submitted papers to the Review committee and to speak with staff and interested persons.

As I had submitted a number of papers from my separate positions of Superintendent of a major Centre, as Past President of the Institute of Ambulance Officers and current Chairman of the Queensland Division, and also as an Interested person, I was ready with substantial evidence to support the introduction of an Ambulance Service administering Emergency Patient Care through certified Officers educated to current standards of Advanced Life Support.

Even so, one had to be very aware and to walk the careful line so as not to expose your intent publicly as there were factions against the Ambulance Service expanding to provide Advanced Emergency Care; others were against the possibility of the Local Committees losing control of the Service even though they themselves had not provided an efficient Service administering a common high standard of Emergency Pre-hospital Patient Care , and there were certain senior Medical Officers within the Health service who were jealously guarding the present control by the Health Department, as to what procedures could be administered by Ambulance Officers.

Why advanced Life Support skills ??
Why should ambulance officers be highly trained ??
Why indeed !

These questions were being asked by a number of people in 1990 because certain academics in the Medical faculty had been touting the pre-hospital care procedure of 'scoop and run' *which, when examined scientifically, was no procedure at all.*

These were mainly a group of Trauma Surgeons and a few Specialists who believed that the only way a victim of road trauma could be 'saved' was for the Ambulance, or any other vehicle, to get that patient to 'a Trauma facility.' Once there one of these Specialist surgeons could 'save' them -- seemingly no one else was capable of this miracle of modern medical science.

My contention was that it was possible to 'get' a road trauma victim to a 'trauma facility' BUT *the victim would not be salvageable if no pre-hospital emergency care had been administered,* and that the time for specialised emergency treatment *was at scene and during transport to definitive medical care* -- therefore suitable officers had to be trained in pre-hospital emergency advanced care.

I had been quietly doing exactly this for some years, educating staff through talks, lectures and correspondence and by training officers to certification standard in ALS with the assistance of Medical Superintendents and Directors of Nursing, particularly at Ipswich.

Some of these advocates for "Scoop and Run" Surgeons had never witnessed the actual and swift deterioration of a trauma patient at scene, and I had to use a graphic description of an actual trauma case where movement of the patient initiated respiratory arrest and on loading into the ambulance, cardiac arrest, to demonstrate the fallacy of this "scoop and run" procedure being advocated.

At the conclusion of my presentation at this meeting of the 'Health and Medical Advisory Committee,' Dr Richard Ashby, Director of the Emergency Department Royal Brisbane Hospital, said "I think we must look at the introduction of intubation by officers in the light of what Malcolm has described."

Support from Medical officers in the direct chain of Emergency care was essential.

Finally the Recommendations from the Select Committee of Inquiry were published and were found to be refreshingly progressive, practicable, and actually sensible, the committee had really listened to officers involved in the Operations of the Service.

The negative side was that the Parliament did not pick up on all the Recommendations and unfortunately did not address those relating to the important financial aspect of supplying a community service.

SOMEONE MUST MAKE THE DECISIONS.

In the present climate of decreed policies of consultation, conciliation and compromise at all costs, this heading could invoke the ire of those who believe in that principle.

It was about a quarter to six, and the chairman of the Ipswich Committee, John Cushing, was discussing the specifications I was drawing up to call quotes for a computer system to suit the growing needs of our establishment.

I had heard some general activity earlier, of phones ringing, doors slamming, and units leaving under power, so I was not surprised when my office phone rang.

" Owen, Super, sorry to disturb you, but we've got a multiple car smash down at Riverview and the primary report says there are six stretcher cases. I've sent three units to scene, but that's all available ....."

" Righto Owen, I'll be down and attend, direct John Hall to the scene, he's on call with 17...."

" Good Super, ah and there's a Doctor at scene."

I turned to the Chairman," want to come?, I'll need a driver on the way back," I said.

Without hesitation John replied," you're on", I grabbed my kit from the shelf, and we hurried down to the plant room, " which unit ?" I asked, as we passed Control," Car one", came the reply.

The adrenalin was flowing, my mind racing, examining the information to hand, the time of day, peak hour traffic from Brisbane, two of our clinic transport buses may be returning also, ten minutes to reach the scene and the injuries had occurred fifteen minutes before now.

Into the old Holden Onetonner Emergency unit, start, lights on, quick check of dash instruments, then gun the motor and out of the centre, siren and flashing red lights.

Acceleration and braking to twist through the streets to the Highway, then flat out towards Riverview, my thoughts on what was before me, any serious patient would be a minimum of twenty five minutes injured by the time we reached the scene.

Good grief!, I remembered something and reached for the radio handset," car 1 to VL4IV ," I called," come in car 1", answered Control.

" Would you notify next door that I am attending, and will be delayed somewhat," I requested.

" Roger car 1," came the answer.

Yes, Control would now inform Val that I was at an emergency and could be delayed for an hour at least.

Val would cease her preparations to attend Rotary Dinner with me that night, and prepare something for our evening meal instead, well that's the ambulance.

All went well until about a kilometre from the scene when we struck a back-up of vehicles clogging the two out lanes; on the other side of the median strip there was heavy inbound traffic.

Off the road and along the water table, I drove, DAMN, a red warning light on the dashboard, we still had 500 metres to go, kept doing, reached the scene.

I stopped the unit, grasped my kit, stepped out, and as I left, I said to John, over my shoulder," she's all yours".

From a distance the scene was pretty with flickering lights, belying the suffering, red, blue and amber, closer it looked chaotic with crashed cars, heavy red Fire units, yellow Ambulances and blue Police cars, and the movement of people.

On scene the movement was controlled and deliberate, with Police directing traffic, protecting the scene, recording statements and co-ordinating any specialised assistance required.

Ambulance officers were treating and removing patients to safety from smashed cars, ready for transport to hospital.

Fire officers were hosing off some leaking petrol, and organising equipment to cut through a car hood to give Ambulance officers access to a trapped patient.

The senior Ambulance officer at scene came to me and gave an update as to number of patients, type of injuries, and officers available.

" Super, there were six stretcher patients, mainly with single injuries, two with a fractured leg, a severe facial laceration, two suspected internal injuries, one of them pregnant, a concussion and one trapped with fractures to both legs and head injury ".

" How bad ? and whose the Doctor ?", I interrupted.

" He's not good, both legs are fractured, one compounded, and he's trapped by the dash at least, a Doctor attached to Commonwealth Health at I.G.H."
" How are we for staff ?", I asked as I turned toward the activity at the one wrecked

car, the report continued.

" The clinic bus returning from Brisbane had stopped, and we loaded two sitting patients who had lacerations, and sent him on his way, and the first Emergency unit has just left with two stretcher cases of suspected internal injuries."

My officer had to talk louder now due to the noise from the generators for the lights, and the diesel motor for the hydraulic cutting equipment.

" There are four Ipswich officers and one from Brisbane, on scene, one with the trapped victim, two splinting the fractures, and myself."

" Right, organise the four stretchers and the sitters into the two emergency units, John Cushing to drive the one with the more serious patients and an officer in the back, the other unit with the conscious less serious patients to only have an officer to drive, get them away as soon as, and ask Control to send the first unit free back to scene", I instructed.

We had arrived at the wrecked car, with the trapped patient who was in a serious condition.

An officer was beside the car, an oxy viva beside him, his head through the window checking the patient, a Fire officer,[his arms full of hydraulic ram and cutting jaws], was about to cut through the last hood strut, two others held the hood from falling onto the patient and the Ambulance officer.

CRACK, and the hood was free, the Firies lifted it up and off the wreck, giving full access to the patient.

" How is he ?," I asked.

The Ambulance officer looked over his shoulder," not the best boss, he's just conscious, but uncooperative, won't tolerate an oxygen mask, has swelling to the side of his head where he's probably hit the windscreen edge, looks like both legs fractured, one compounded, can feel the blood, and trapped by the dash at least", came the full report.

" Right, we'll get a collar on him, and get some obs recorded."

The Fire Brigade Station officer saw me and came around, "we'll pull the dash forward, if that's O'k with you, and then see what else is in the road," he said.

"That seems right to me Officer", I answered," carry on, I'll ask if there's anything we want done".

I saw the Doctor approaching, by the badge of office, the stethoscope at her neck, and I picked up the portable radio,
" 4IV, Super here", I called. "Control to Superintendent", was the answer.

" Control, the site is under control, but we have a trapped patient in a serious condition, I want Senior officer Hall in the new Modular Unit as soon as, call him and check his position please," as I clicked to 'receive' John came on the air, " car 17 approaching Riverview now, over."

Beaut! I needed the large Modular unit, it's equipment, and John's certified skills.

"4IV Superintendent to Car 17, attend as close to the Fire Rescue Unit as possible for access to the patient, over," I called, forestalling Control, " Roger, car 1", John replied.

The Doctor was beside us now, so I gave her the report on our patient, ending with - “the Modular Emergency unit with full resuscitation gear will be on scene within minutes, with an officer certified for cannulation and assistance with intubation - this is available for your use."

"Thank you," was the courteous reply.

We checked the patient, he had deteriorated a little, he was presenting early symptoms of shock, still un-cooperative, barely conscious, I was concerned at his condition and the prolonged extrication required.

I instructed my officer to persist with oxygen therapy, even though the patient pushed the mask away.

Car 17 arrived and was positioned close to us.

The Fire officers had fitted a chain and hook to the dash and applied leverage to pull it forward, but the patient was still trapped by his legs from the seat edge and front fire wall, some time yet to have him free.

I went to Car 17 and spoke to Senior officer Hall," John, I want you to prepare a unit of Haemacell with a giving set, and a wide bore needle, this patient will need access for drug therapy or fluid replacement or both, the Doctor will decide, but get it ready now."

Officer Bennett had appeared from somewhere, so I asked him to bring a stretcher over to the trapped patient.

I returned to the trapped patient.

The Brisbane officer arrived with an Ipswich officer who reported, "all other patients have been treated and transported from scene Super."

"Well done," I replied almost subconsciously, because the patient had lost consciousness, the Fire officers were working to cut away the seat supports to free his fractured legs, so he could be lifted out.

The unconscious patient cried out and rolled his head from side to side, a sign of brain irritation.

Time for hard decisions, "support his head, and maintain his airway!" to the Brisbane officer, "Bob when he is out and in the unit, you will splint his legs, John(Bennett) you will apply oxygen therapy and airway management."

"Stop the extrication", I ordered," he's coming out now."

The Fire officers 'looked' the question, but stopped.

This was no time for consultation, time was of the essence.

Senior officer Hall walked over.

" John! I'll pull his legs free, organise officers to lift him out by his shoulders and then his waist, supporting him full length as he comes out, you know, our a caterpillar lift."

John didn't need telling, we had devised this extrication procedure to protect a patient from further injury and used it before, only this time I could cause some pain at least, as I twisted his fractured legs free.

" Lift " I instructed, and as the patient was lifted off the seat, I grasped one leg and pulled it free of the wreckage, then pulled the other fractured leg free, which was easier due to being compounded.

I heard John calmly commanding the lift and move ," steady chaps, keep him level, support that leg now, righto lower gently, well done, into the unit now,"

The Doctor and I moved to the unit," John can cannulate, if you wish Doctor," I indicated.

" Yes, I'd like a unit of fluid put up and run to keep his veins open and available for Casualty, and transported as soon as possible."

The officers were working as a team, the compound fractured leg had a splint in place and was being bandaged, John Hall had the cannula inserted, so I quickly stepped into the back and taped the needle in place as he connected the drip tube and ran the fluid, officer Bennett had the oxygen therapy mask in place and oxygen flowing.

I looked at the Doctor, she nodded," leave the other leg ",I instructed, " let's go."

The patient was transported to Ipswich General Hospital, and due to early notification to the Hospital of the patient's condition, a Hospital team was waiting.

A quick but expert examination of the patient in Casualty department, drugs into the 'line', then an immediate continuation to theatre where the Surgeon drilled a burr hole to relieve the intracranial pressure from the internal haemorrhage.

Further surgery followed to set the compound fracture, then a period of nursing care.

Due to the concerted effort by all members of the Health team the patient made a full recovery, and was discharged from hospital carrying a number of scars but well and healthy.

I thought the job had been managed very professionally, but my satisfaction was somewhat spoiled a few weeks later when, as the 'Boss', I received a phone call complaining about the Ambulance account, on the grounds that the patient had not asked for an Ambulance.

This type of complaint unfortunately is not strange to us, the Ambulance can do everything in it's power to administer to a patient but receive no thanks, and even, as in this case, receive criticism and complaint - **YOU CAN'T WIN 'EM ALL.**

IT MUST BE LEGAL – THE FORCES MUSTER.

1991 - THE BUREAU OF EMERGENCY SERVICES.

The Government formed the Bureau of Emergency Services with Police, Fire and SES services and with the intent for the Ambulance to join.

The Minister for Emergency Services was the Hon. Terry Mackenroth, MLA. and the Director General of Emergency Services was Mr. Howard Baker.

Over a few years before the formation of the Bureau of Emergency Services I had written to the appropriate Ministers advocating the introduction of:-
Advanced Life Support procedures,
Pre-hospital coronary care,
Control of the patient 'at scene'
The Ambulance to remain a separate Emergency Service.

On the formation of the infant Bureau of Emergency Services, [before the Ambulance was committed], I wrote to the Director General submitting the Structure for a State Emergency Service and on various initiatives.

These representations must have established my credibility for I was appointed by the Minister as the Co-ordinator of the Legislation Task Force to write the Ambulance Services Act - 1991, and also co-ordinator of the Task Force to write the Operational Standards and Protocol manual for the new Service - *a challenge and we had to triumph.*

MINISTER FOR POLICE AND EMERGENCY SERVICES

The Hon. Terry Mackenroth M.P.
Member for Chatsworth

20th March, 1991

Mr M. McDonald
Superintendent
Q.A.T.B. Ipswich
P.O. Box 408
IPSWICH. Q. 4305

Dear Mr McDonald,

As you are aware Cabinet considered the recommendations of the Parliamentary Select Committee of Inquiry into Ambulance Services' report and has accepted a number of recommendations.

Enclosed are copies of the summary of recommendations of the Parliamentary Select Committee and Cabinet's position on the major recommendations for your information.

In order to create the Queensland Ambulance Service and effect the legislative, structural and operational changes required by 1st July, 1991, a Committee system has been established. This Committee structure is also attached for your information.

I invite you to attend a full day seminar on Wednesday, 27th March, 1991 commencing 9.00 a.m. at the David Muir Room, Floor 2, Education House, 30 Mary Street, Brisbane as Co-ordinator of the Legislation Task Force and the Operational Standards and Protocol Task Force.

The purpose of the seminar is to commence implementation of Cabinet's decision to re-organise Queensland's Ambulance Service. A program for the seminar will be forwarded to you in due course.

This is an exciting time for Queensland's Ambulance Service and I appreciate your participation in this major project.

I look forward to seeing you on the 27th March, 1991.

Yours sincerely,

TERRY MACKENROTH
Minister for Police and
Emergency Services

POSTAL: G.P.O. Box 1425, Brisbane, 4001. OFFICE: 31st Floor, M.L.C. Centre, 239 George Street, Brisbane, 4000.
TELEPHONE: (07) 227 4910 FACSIMILE: (07) 221 9042

Ministerial Task Force members:

LEGISLATION TASK FORCE

Co-ordinator:	M. McDonald, Superintendent/Secretary, QATB Ipswich Committee R.S. Forbes, Assistant Manager, Queensland Ambulance Services Board N. Rees, Federated Miscellaneous Workers Union
Parliamentary Counsel Liaison Officer:	Wayne Ripper, Bureau of Emergency Services (P. Young, Advisor)

ORGANISATION STRUCTURE AND INDUSTRIAL RELATIONS TASK FORCE

Co-ordinator:	J. McPherson, Superintendent/Secretary, QATB Brisbane Committee B. Toogood, Superintendent/Secretary, QATB Innisfail Committee B. Daly, Accountant, Queensland Ambulance Services Board I. Shakespeare, Industrial Officer, QASB for Industrial Relations matters J. Slowgrove, Federated Miscellaneous Workers Union S. Crow, Ambulance Officer, QATB Brisbane Committee R. Simpson, Principal Consultant, Bureau of Emergency Services

FUNDING AND BUDGET TASK FORCE

Co-ordinator:	B. Daly, Accountant, Queensland Ambulance Services Board R. Singh, Superintendent/Secretary, QATB Mareeba Committee R. Lackey, Superintendent/Secretary, QATB Charters Towers Committee P. Mitchell, Administration Officer, QATB Rockhampton Committee D. Bray, Assistant Director, Administration and Finance, Bureau of Emergency Services

OPERATIONAL STANDARDS AND PROTOCOL TASK FORCE

Co-ordinator	M. McDonald, Superintendent, QATB Ipswich Committee L. Wilson, Deputy Superintendent, QATB Brisbane Committee M.A. Ollis, Training Officer, QATB Clermont Committee T. Tighe, Assistant Inspector of Committees, Queensland Ambulance Services Board

SACRIFICE FOR POLITICAL EXPEDIENCY - 3 months to do it all.

The Minister for Police and Emergency Services, the Hon. Terry Mackenroth, appointed his Task Force co-ordinators on the 20th. March and called them to their first meeting for the 27th. March 1991, but this was held the next day, the 28th.

The Minister informed the Task Force Co-ordinators that they were expected to carry out their brief by the 1st.July 1991 so that the new Queensland Ambulance Service could commence operations - 3 months to complete the total restructuring of the State Ambulance Service - some job.

The Legislation Task Force was the only Task Force which did not have the full 3 months. The timeframe given us was:
We had to draft the Legislation, have the draft Bill written, consult with all Government Departments, have the Draft Bill accepted by all involved Departments and in the Cabinet Bag in sufficient time for 'approval,' then time to Introduce the 'Bill' to become an Act, to be 'passed,' and finally Proclaimed for commencement by July 1.

For without "The Ambulance Service Act," the new State Ambulance Service could not come into being, and that would be a political disaster.

It was a major task, as it rested on my ability to control the evolution of the final Bill so that it reflected all the salient requirements, regulations and legalities for the conduct of an Ambulance Service which would deliver a high standard of Emergency and Pre-Hospital care, and to provide staff and patient protection.

My other task of writing the Operational Standards and Protocol manual was almost as important, as these were also required to be written, printed and distributed to every Station in Queensland by the 1st.July 1991, so that all Stations would operate as a co-ordinated State Service.

I called the Operational Standards and Protocol Task Force together and we discussed the urgent need for a common set of Operational Procedures to be in place by 1st July 1991.

I spoke of the need for clear, practical and professional content as this would set the standard for the future delivery of our Service to Queensland.
I briefly outlined the established MOP used by Ipswich District as it encompassed the Pre-hospital Emergency care system.

I set them to examining Ipswich and Brisbane MOP, to select procedural clauses common to both and for specific sections addressing Emergency procedures for examination at our next meeting.
This gave me time to devote to the Legislation Task Force.

I was able to devote my full attention to this Task Force after May 14th.

This Task force edited the Manual, item by item, page after page, and there was some lively discussion as to meaning and interpretation.
We had the volume of Operational Standards and Protocol written and approved by the Steering Committee to print.

I personally called on the Printer amongst his presses, who was to actually "print" the manual, and discussed the essential need for the Manuals to be 'out' by 1.7.1991. Even though he had a heavy commitment of work to Government Departments, he accepted the urgency for publication and I received his full cooperation and he delivered on time.

One copy of the MOP was distributed to every Station in Queensland in the first week of July 1991.
This was followed by further copies for all staff.

Due to the rather hurried drafting and expected changes to the Service, *I gave a proviso that the Operational Procedures should be reviewed within 6 months.*

Other Task Forces such as the Organisation Structure and Industrial Relations Task Force were still deliberating as to final decisions after the Act had been proclaimed and after the new QAS had commenced.

I was still Superintendent of the Ipswich District responsible for the administration and Operations of the Ambulance Service within that large area, but daily meetings in Brisbane and the time required to research and write presentations for the two Task Forces as well as the resulting minutes took many hours of the day.

To ensure an efficient service I appointed my Deputy, John Hall, to carry out the general responsibilities of Superintendent with the appropriate salary and conditions, and I took a supervisory role only.

As the 1st of July approached I was appointed interim Deputy Commissioner, Planning and Support services, so I was now fully occupied in the establishment of the QAS.
I was still on my Superintendent's wage paid by the Ipswich Centre Committee, all of the work and hours expended for the formation of the new QAS was from commitment and loyalty to the Service.

As a spare time activity I was the Chairman of the International Conference on Pre-hospital Emergency Care to be held in October 1992, this had been initiated from Ipswich two years previously under the auspices of the Institute of Ambulance Officers of Australia, so that took care of any time left in the 24 hour day.

THE WRITING OF THE AMBULANCE SERVICE ACT - 1991.

As I had given much thought, over a period of time, to the need for certain requirements to be included in any new Act, and made a number of submissions to the Minister on the proposed Service, I was well prepared, experienced, and knowledgeable for the task, in fact there was no other person in Queensland who could equal my Ambulance qualifications and operational experience, and my record of presentation of Papers on various aspects of Ambulance Pre-hospital Emergency Care and Procedures at Medical Conferences.

Members of the Legislation Task force were :-

Legislation Co-ordinator.	: Malcolm McDonald, Fellow Institute Ambulance Officers (Aust.), Superintendent Ipswich Ambulance District; QATB Operational qualifications to Coronary Care.
Parliamentary Council Liaison officer.	: Wayne Ripper, Public Service Admin officer.
Legislation Advisor	: Peter Young, Cabinet Legislation and Liaison Officer
Qld. Ambulance Services Board,	
QASB	: Bob Forbes, administration officer.
State Union	: Norm Reece , FMWU representative.

As appointed Co-ordinator, I conducted the meetings and recorded the business of the meetings as a confidential Minute, and submitted a Report to each meeting of the Steering Committee.

On my Report being accepted by the Steering Committee, the relevant proposals/amendments were directed to the Drafting Solicitor M. Mc Garry, Crown Solicitor, who then prepared these, [progressively], into legal form as a Draft section of the 'Act.'

This draft was then submitted by hand to the Parliamentary Counsel Vince Hebbard.

The task of Parliamentary Counsel was to attend to the intent of the clauses, to check the legal correctness of each draft, and to ensure that the content did not contravene or contradict ANY other Act.
He would then amend/rewrite the Draft where necessary and return these recommendations to the Task Force.

When I closed the first meeting of the Legislation Task Force, the Parliamentary Counsel Liaison Officer informed the meeting that my minutes of the meeting would be provided to the Drafting Solicitor for compilation into Draft form for the final Bill which would then be presented to Parliamentary Counsel by himself and the Drafting Solicitor.

I could see shades of Public Service ineptitude, so I put to the Task Force that as Co-ordinator and the only qualified Operational Officer on the committee, I should be included in any meeting with the Parliamentary Counsel.
As there was no valid reason for my not being present, this was resolved, and I attended at every meeting with the Parliamentary Counsel.

Without my insistence of being present at the meetings with Parliamentary Counsel there would have been a very different Ambulance Services Act, one that was much weaker in substance and one that would have left the Ambulance Service as a poor relation to the other Emergency Service members and to the Public Service.

I had thought out the necessary items to be included in the Act and these had to be interwoven into the different sections, in this would be their strength.
This all pivoted in the wording of the definitions at the very commencement of the Act.

Peter Young, Advisor, and the Cabinet Legislation and Liaison Officer, ensured the integrity of the documents, then their movement from the Task force, through the Minister's office, then on to the Parliamentary Counsel and back to me.

The timeframe to meet the deadline for passage as a 'Bill' was Peter's responsibility.

The Public Service Order:
The Parliamentary Counsel was an extremely important and busy person, so we three from Legislation had to meet with him after 5.30pm when he had concluded his more pressing business for the day.

Parliamentary Counsel sat behind his desk. 'We three' sat in a row in front of the desk, diligently alert.

The Counsel Liaison Officer would put forward the Draft Act items under discussion, and provide an explanation of same:
- the Parliamentary Counsel would read this and might ask a question –
- one of 'we three' would answer.

Counsel would then make a pertinent comment – *and presumably by Public Service protocol, the two Public servants would defer to this.*
I was not a Public servant, so I was free to comment when I believed an incorrect definition was put forward.
I would respectfully give the Ambulance Operational meaning or explanation which was often contrary to the natural and researched conclusion drawn by the Parliamentary Counsel, as his decision as to wording had to consider ALL other Acts.
Draft Act – items 1 to 4:

THE 'OLD' AND THE 'NEW' ACT.

As Co-ordinator addressing the content of the new act, my areas of concern were:-
The old Act defined Ambulance Service as 'transport of the sick and injured,' and to 'render first aid.' This had to change to reflect current techniques & treatments.

The first major difference was in the old definition of "Ambulance Service" being '**the rendering of First aid etc.**' and the difference ***with my definition of 'Emergency treatment and Pre-hospital patient care.'***

The Parliamentary Counsel then questioned me as to the meaning and implications of my point, because as he said, "**it was previously 'First Aid' and other States had the wording as 'First aid'**."
The Task Force Convenor explained that the **QAS provided Basic Life Support (BLS) and Advanced Life Support (ALS)** as compared to **First aid by St. John and laypersons etc.**
That 'First-aid' was defined as 'initial care' in the St. John text book, and 'Medical aid' as that received from a Doctor, an R.N., or Ambulance officer.
The Parliamentary Counsel agreed to include this. ref: diary & Task Force papers.

The Parliamentary Counsel listened as I explained the progress we had made in the delivery of Pre-hospital Care and gave me the respect of my position. He redrafted the clause to give this contemporary definition of our operational role.
This was the pattern of our future meetings. He would look to me for Operational advice or for explanation of a particular point, and might or might not amend some wording of a particular clause.

I found him to show dignified understanding, and to be a most expert and articulate gentleman.
Some points discussed:
The Ambulance Service had little input into actual Counter Disaster planning and in Patient care, and little authorised control over the patient generally in this situation.
<u>Another concern in relation to Search and Rescue</u> was the initial assessment of the casualty/patient, and the possibility of incorrect management of the patient by unskilled/inexperienced people which could either delay correct treatment or cause further injury
<u>At the accident or emergency scene</u>, volunteer groups such as Mines Rescue, St. John Ambulance, Railway Ambulance Corps, Scouts and Guides were each under their own command and independent of any official direction from the Ambulance Service, thus allowing for confusion and conflicting procedures for patient management.

The Ambulance officer had no legal rights for entry to the locked premises of an injured or ill patient, nor at the scene of violent or potentially violent behaviour.

The proliferation of teaching techniques and procedures in First-aid which were not always in co-ordination with the procedures for Emergency Pre-hospital Patient Care as practised by the Ambulance Service, the then QATB.

To announce any action to countermand any one of these jealously guarded power bases would have caused an immediate and powerful reaction, with self interest rather than patient-interest to the fore.
So I kept the overall strategy to myself and officially dealt with each issue as a separate item, outwardly giving such items no importance individually but privately ensuring each fitted in the overall plan, for taken as a whole they constituted a major shift in giving the authority and control to the Ambulance Service for the care of all casualties/patients.

After numerous meetings and appearances before the Steering Committee 'the Act' was drafted, well, there was a number of 'drafts.'

I had walked the minefield, there had been a few eruptions, some losses, but mainly success in maintaining the integrity of 'The Act' to ensure the Ambulance was a Service relating to the work of rendering emergency treatment and pre-hospital patient care to, and the transport of, sick and injured persons.

In brief, the functions of the Queensland Ambulance Service as defined:-
to provide an Ambulance service and during rescue and other related activities, to protect persons from injury or death, whether or not those persons are sick or injured. To participate with other Emergency services in Counter Disaster planning and to coordinate all volunteer first aid groups in respect of major emergencies or disasters. To provide casualty room services and to provide community and workplace education in First-aid, cardiopulmonary resuscitation and other related matters.
In between Task Force and Steering Committee meetings, I was 'called in' by DBES Howard Baker as he received 'briefs' from the various Departments for either support or inquiry. One such demanded a meeting with Health Department Officers who were concerned as to certain clause re the transport of patients within Hospital grounds and other related situations. This meeting required my attendance and the discussion was rather robust but courteous, resulting in a mutual change in wording.

The Legislation Task Force first met at an introductory meeting on 28th March 1991 to commence the drafting of The Bill, which would became The Act, in time for all legal requirements to be met for it to be in force to allow the commencement of the new Queensland Ambulance Service.

We had the Bill in the Cabinet Bag on 14.5.1991 - in 46 days.
This was slightly behind the timetable but in ample time for the Act to be in force on the 1st.July 1991

I believe that the combined efforts of all members orchestrated an Act which encompassed all the necessary criteria, safeguards and authority for the conduct of a contemporary Ambulance Service of a high standard.

I was, and am, proud to have been a major part of the formulation of "The Ambulance Service Act 1991."

Of course, a number of political changes have been made to the Act over a period which allowed for one major change I had initiated to be realised.
In June of 1991 the Ipswich Ambulance commenced a Pre-hospital Emergency Care Trial for the intravenous cannulation of patients requiring fluid replacement / infusion therapy for particular medical conditions.

Specific Pre-hospital Care patients would receive "A Shot in the Arm."

Ipswich Centre advised certain Centres on the Procedure to follow and supplied QATB Ipswich Training notes and slides to support the introduction of this lifesaving procedure.

On the 30th June 1991 I ceased as Superintendent of Ipswich Ambulance District to take up the interim position of Deputy Commissioner Planning and Support and we moved from our residence of twelve and a half years at the Ambulance Centre, to our own home at Mooloolah on two and a half acres on the Ewan Maddock Dam.

It was a sad parting for we had made many friends in Ipswich and had worked with many people to upgrade the Ambulance Service and other services in that district.
I continued in my spare time activity as Chairman of the International Conference on Pre-hospital Emergency Care to be held in October 1992.
This had been initiated from Ipswich two years previously under the auspices of the Institute of Ambulance Officers of Australia.

But the incessant demand upon me from early in 1991, in the first instance from the Director General of the Bureau of Emergency Services to attend meeting with him discussing submissions and attending preliminary meetings with Health and Public Service officers.

Then from the Minister with Legislation, still with the responsibilities as Superintendent of Ipswich Centre until July, followed by six months duties of Interim Deputy Commissioner Planning and Support Services.

In the first instance the Public Service provided no assistance in regard to Administration manuals and support information relevant to the changeover process.
The continuous demand on my services caused an insidious deterioration to my general health.

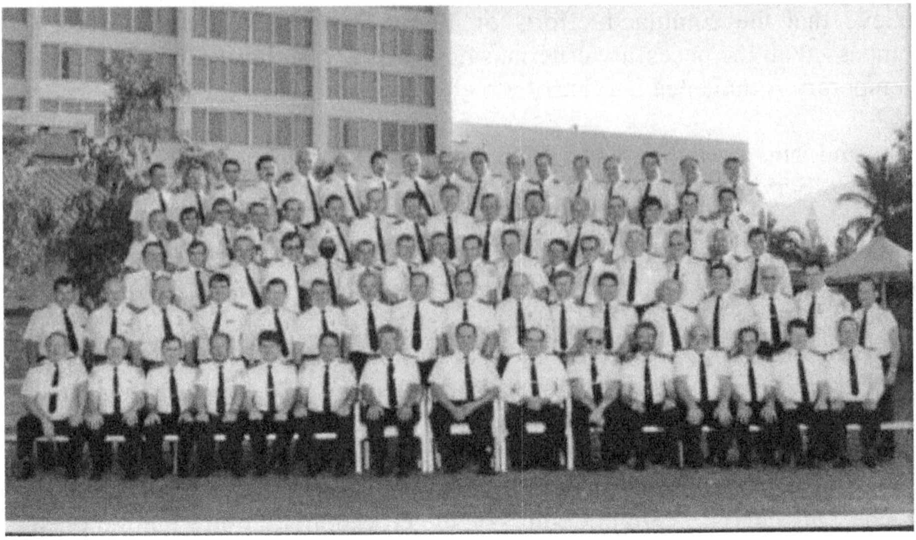

QATB Superintendents 1991.

Superintendents
QATB State Conference - Townsville 1989

Back Row:	Len *PRICE* (Laidley);	Terry *BOYD* (Gladstone);	Ron *FLETCHER (Mt Morgan)*;	Tim *IRVING* (Injune);
	Allan G0TTKE (Cooroy);	Kevin *TOOTEL* (Mundubbera);	Trevor *TIGHE* (Gayndah);	Kent *LARSEN* (Clifton);
	Ben *CLUTTERBUCK* (Childers);	David *TREVOR* (Springsure);	Henry *WEEKS* (Coolangatta);	Ian *HALLIWELL (Charleville)*;
	Maurie *SWEEDMAN* (Miles);	Merv *LUCUS* (Atherton);	John *NICHOLSON* (Home Hill);	Robert *MACKNEY (Roma)*.
	Brian *MOORE* (Beaudesert).			
Forth Row:	Cecil *KRISANSKI* (Toogoolawah);	Dennis *GILL* (Monto);	Rick *LEONARD* (St George);	Allan *BROWN* (Caboolture);
	Rod *SHEATHER* (Yarraman);	Vic *TORRENS* (Stanthorpe);	Mick *O'MARA (Pittsworth)*;	John *McLENNAN* (Maleny);
	Hugh *BARCLAY* (Caloundra);	Fred *FREEMAN* (Texas);	Robert *LACKEY* (Charters Towers);	Robert *WARNOCK* (Hervey Bay);
	Philip *CRAWFORD* (Emerald);	John *MOYNIHAM* (Julia Creek);	Graham *BECKER* (Taroom);	Robert *McILROY* (Blackall)
Third Row:	Richie *OLIVERI* (Ingham);	Trevor *HALLEWELL* (Kilcoy);	Ron *JAMES* {Mossman};	Malcolm *HAMPSON* (Mt Isa);
	Resham *SINGH* (Mareeba);	Noel *PEGG* {Boonah};	Colin *McKAY*(Rockhampton);	Ray *TRENAMAN* (Mackay);
	Geoff *VENZ* (Nambour);	Carl *COLEMAN* {Bowen};	Peter *FOX* (Cloncurry);	*Cecil BUTLER* (Kinaroy);
	Raymond *NEWITT* (Warwick);	Mick *MILLER* (St George);	Geoffrey *JOHNSTONE* (Yeppoon);	Raymond *GREENWOOD* (Proston).
Second Row:	Geoffrey *REYNOLDS* (Cairns);	Reg *BRENNAN* (Biloela);	Philip *MOORE* (Wynnum);	Gregory *HARDY* (Mt Larcom);
	Leo *McNAMIARA* (Millmerran);	Neville *CHURCH* (Oaky);	Ralph *EAGLE (Tully)*;	Graham *SEALY* (Hughendon);
	Wally WARRENER (Biggendon);	Robert *TUTTLE* (Clermont);	Patrick *DENHAM* (Proserpine);	Lindsay *ROBERTS* (Rosewood);
	Keith *SMITH* (Mungon);	Gary *GREENHILL* (Winton);	Lino *BAGAROZZA* (Bundeberg);	Robert *MEDLIN* (Ravenshoe);
	Gordon *KRAUSE* (Dayboro).			
Front Row:	Barry *BRYANT* (Beenleigh);	Ronald *LAWRENCE (Gympie)*.	Edward *ROBERTSON* (Gordanvale);	Trevor *SKINNER* (Collinsville);
	Stephen *BURNS* (Wowan);	Gary *BURROWS* (Surat);	Desmond *CONDON* (Townsville);	John *McPHERSON* (Brisbane);
	Robert *HASWELL* (Toowoomba);	John *KLOHS* (Ayr);	Stephen *ALLEN* (Dirranbandi);	Ted *SHEPHERD* (Thursday Isle).
	Robert *PRATT* (Redlands);	Malcolm *McDONALD*	Bert *TOOGOOD* (Innisfail).	*81 pictured*
Not Pictured:	Greg *BALINT* (Aramac)	Wally *BUCKLEY* (Baralaba)	V C *KENNETT* (Chinchilla)	W *COLLINS* (Goondiwindi)
	W F *FISHER* (Dalby)	G E *SCHMIERER* (Gatton)	R L R *DAVIS* (Gin Gin)	R *BAILEY* (Inglewood)
	Rod *MULLER* (Millaa Millaa)	L F *LEWINGTON* (Mitchell)	G *SKERMAN* (Mount Garnet)	K J *CUSKELLY* (Nanango)
	Allan *GOTTKE* (Noosa)	Syd *CROSS* (Southport)	Gordon *BRYANT* (Theordore)	*13 non pictured*

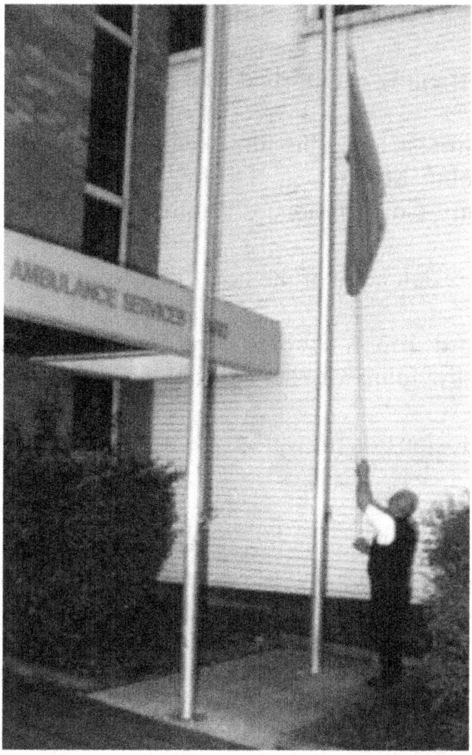

THE LAST and THE FIRST DAYS:

THE CLOSING OF AN ERA – the QATB flag is lowered on the 28th June 1991

THE QAS 1991 – 2016.

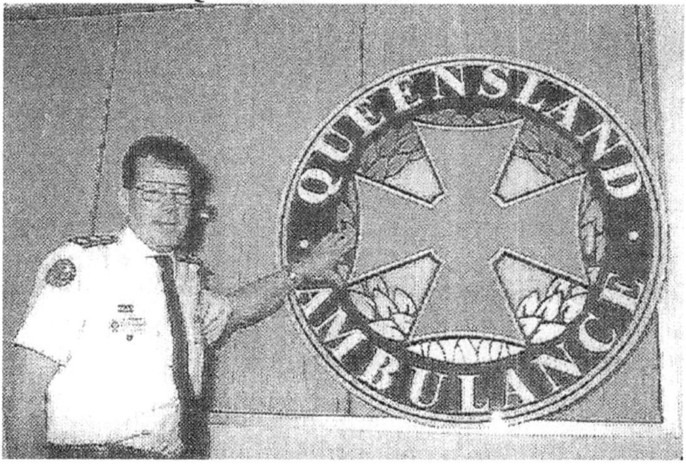

Demonstration of the first QAS LOGO design to identify the new service.

1st JULY 1991 – A NEW DAY AND A NEW SERVICE BEGINS

On this day the new QAS structure was officially established as a Division of The Bureau of Emergency Services.
The interim appointments had been made in respect of the most senior QATB staff. Dr. Gerry FitzGerald Commissioner, John McPherson Deputy Commissioner Operations and Malcolm McDonald Deputy Commissioner Planning and Support Services.
So here we were on July 1st. 1991, the first official day of the new QAS.

I well remember walking into the Board room of the previous Queensland Ambulance Services Board, now shared by John McPherson and myself as our temporary office for the past few weeks.
It was 7am, but there was no colourful explosions of fireworks, there were no Bands playing, it was simply quiet and isolated.

The long table, which had previously experienced luminaries of the President of the QASB and Chairman of QATB Committees sitting around its impressive length, deciding the fate of the Queensland service, now stood isolated with only 2 chairs at one side. Portable phones for both John and I in the centre with neat stacks of folders and files at each end.
No secretarial staff – just us AND the Public Service.

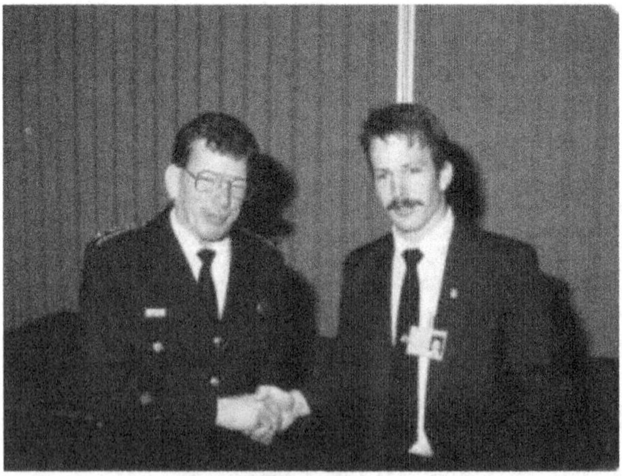

But, first things first – it was the first day of the **QAS Associate Diploma Course.**

The interim Commissioner Dr. Gerald FitzGerald and the Deputy Commissioner Planning and Support were on their way to Ipswich for the Commissioner to officially introduce the QAS Associate Diploma Course and to welcome the first students.

Interim Deputy Commissioner Planning and Support welcomes Mark McDonald CTS Resource Officer as the Co-ordinator of the QAS Associate Diploma Course.

I will provide the actual conditions and problems of the earliest days of establishing co-ownership of the QAS with the departments of the Public service.

The Act had been written, but the full recommendations of the Select Committee of Inquiry had not been approved by Parliament.

Hard issues such as Finance had been left as a 'part government- part subscription/charge' with no real strategy to finance this new service.

The Government of the day had been given the uninformed advice *that the restructuring of the QATB to the QAS as a State body could be carried out at neutral cost, ie without any increase in funding from the Government.*

On that day all QATB Committees ceased to exist and the new QAS become responsible for the provision of all Ambulance Services throughout Queensland and responsible for all vehicles, equipment, buildings and the training of all staff, *ie* for 96 Ambulance stations throughout Queensland, *and now responsible for any problems or complaints state-wide.*

So here we were with no official office, no official secretary, no filing cabinets nor filing system, no administration manual, but being experienced Ambulance Officers faced with problems we improvised and delivered.

The new Act had been drafted in time for it to be in force on the 1st July.
The Operational Procedures for the delivery of Service and the direction of the 'on-road' staff was completed and printed with a copy at each station on the 1st.July.
BUT, the organizational structure had not been finalized nor was there any administration manual available for us as was used by the Public servants who formed the Corporate Administration body of the Emergency Services structure!!

We were interim Deputy Commissioners and we and the system were in total transitional mode.

About mid July we moved into the Bureau of Emergency Services Headquarters in Forbes House opposite the Police Headquarters, with our offices on the 10th floor. The Minister was on the 13th floor - yes it might have been prophetic as we had 4 Ministers from the Labor Government in the 2 years 1991-1993.

The blatant questions which required direct answers were:-
What was Corporate Services responsibility and what was the QAS Executives' responsibility? Who was to direct the finances? *Oh that was the job of Treasury!*

It was Treasury who had advised the Minister that the change from the QATB Committee system to the state QAS would be financially neutral!!

This in itself showed a lack of accountability to say the least.
This set the greatest problem which was to plague us and which caused the greatest confusion and retardation of the QAS in this introductory stage.
The contributions and accounts were in disarray for 6 months.

And the Corporate Services costs went up and UP and UP.

Yes, we became enmeshed in the quagmire of Bureaucratic policies and political machinations to deflect responsibility.
For someone who was used to making instant decisions and being responsible for his actions and in control of such actions, this was more than frustrating and I was to feel this even more as time went on and politics interfered more in the decision making process.
We are now working out of the BES headquarters, which was a vast improvement as we were allocated offices to our station with secretarial staff.

There is little time for consolidation, to settle into a cohesive team, but decisions had to be made.

What's that? another meeting to attend, can't we just get on with the implementation of the new Service?
OH! It's from 'Treasury' on 'Future Planning and the development of Strategies' - but I thought we had just done all of that over the 3 months with the various Task Forces ? - right! the memo from the Director states a member of senior staff shall attend, and I'm the lesser of the three - O'K.

Memo from the Minister's office:- a meeting on 'Women's rights in the Workplace' at 9am and a Senior Executive officer from all Divisions of the Bureau will attend - well that's me alright.

Another first - *The dreaded red folder from the Minister's office - a Ministerial!*

'the Minister requires a briefing on this matter before Parliaments sits at 2pm.' - but it's 11am now !
Wait a moment, by the date stamps on the folder it's been up THERE for two weeks already!! all right, all right, I'll leave what I'm doing and investigate and write a reply immediately.

We had arrived at last, *the QAS was now a part of the Bureaucratic Grand Design* and we *were only beginning to learn all about it.*

Then came combined District meetings, Regional meetings, Executive meetings, Bureau meetings, meetings to decide when to have a meeting, *no time for our core role of management.*

Due to years of administrative experience the Queensland Ambulance Service continued to operate despite the Bureaucratic jungle growing unchecked, but we were all subject to the Public Service expertise of containment.

The Commissioner of the Queensland Ambulance Service was appointed in late August 1991.

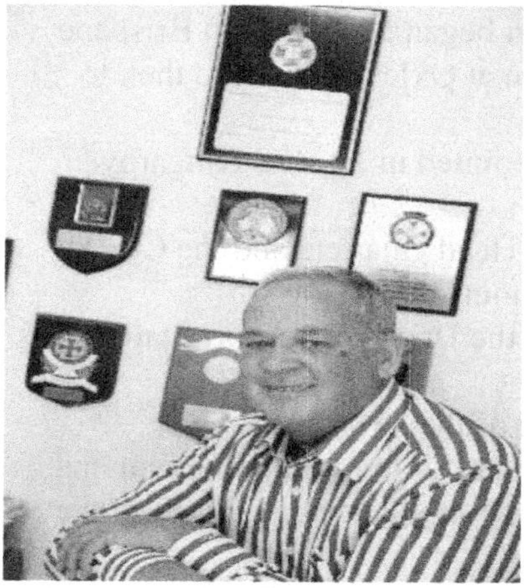

First Commissioner QAS: Noel Gillard, OAM.

An ambulance officer for 25 years before taking up education and executive roles.

Superintendent of the Tasmanian Ambulance Service until 1989 when he was appointed Ambulance Director of the ACT Service.

In 1991 Noel was appointed as Commissioner of the new Queensland Ambulance Service and retired in 2011.

Noel has been an Officer in St. John Ambulance for many years.

A Fellow of the IAO(Aust.) and Chair of the Education Committee, Noel had a long involvement with the Institute and served a term as President.

The positions for Deputy Commissioners had been called and interviews were conducted after the appointment of the Commissioner in late August, BUT it took 3 months before the appointees were decided and announced.
It seems that an outside choice had been made which was finally proven to be unsound, so further behind-the-scene moves and counter moves took place until appointments were finally made.

QAS SENIOR ADMINISTRATION APPOINTED:

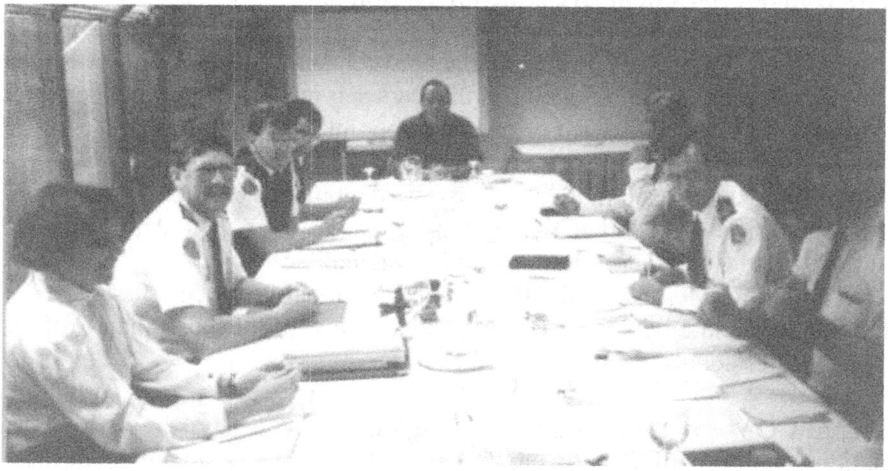

QAS 1991 – Management profiles taken from a QAS press release:

Deputy Commissioner Kenneth John McPherson began as an A/O in Brisbane for two years followed by a permanent staff position at Oxley sub-centre then to Thursday Is in 1966.
John spent the next three years at Theodore and appointed in 1974 to Kingaroy before final posting at Rockhampton in 1981.
During this term of office John supervised the new Head Quarters and the CQ Air Ambulance Service three planes, six pilots and 24 hours on the job.
Appointed as Superintendent of Brisbane in 1989 - the Brisbane Airport Station was opened under his tenure.
John McPherson had an involvement with planning of the new QAS.
He was President of the Superintendents Association prior to his appointment and brought an extensive appreciation of every aspect of Ambulance operations to the Service.

Deputy Commissioner Planning and Support Services Peter McMurtrie.
Peter comes to Queensland via the Goulburn Valley after his term as area Superintendent Metropolitan. He had serious experience in Major Disasters.

Peter has had extensive experience in all ambulance operations including Training and air ambulance. He served for ten years as a State Emergency Service Controller and membership of the Australian IAO, the Australian Management Institute and the Australian Resuscitation Council. He is also qualified in Health services management.
This experience will stand in good for the rigors of his new posting.

THE ASSISTANT COMMISSIONERS:

Malcolm McDonald, A-Com at Brisbane for Region 5.
Malcolm McDonald's ambulance career began in 1955 as an Honorary at Cairns, AO in western Qld at Julia Creek, Air Ambulance Attendant in Rockhampton Central Qld Aerial Ambulance and includes 22 years service as a Superintendent at Wowan, Maleny, Gatton and Ipswich prior to his appointment in 1991.
Malcolm developed the Ipswich Emergency Pre-hospital Care System and the introduction of intravenous cannulation infusion by Ambulance Officers at scene.
He was Convener of the Legislative Task Force for the writing of The Ambulance Service Act 1991 and Convener of the Procedure Manual.
Malcolm is a Founding Member of the IOA(Aust.), National President 1984 and Chairman of Queensland Division up to 1991 and a Fellow of the Australian College of Ambulance Professionals

Allen Marr, A. COM. at Toowoomba, for Region 3.
Congratulations on his appointment were the order of the day from members of the IAO, from his position as National secretary immediately before his appointment. A career start in the Victorian service in 1969 led to qualifications as an AO and transfer to Mildura two years later.

On his next appointment as SO at Hastings Branch, he attended nearly 200 flights as an attendant on the "Angel of Mercy" helicopter based nearby. SSO at Echuca until 1988 when at Regionalisation he moved to Swan Hill as District Superintendent in charge of the Mallee District.
Allen believes strongly that ambulance officers should enjoy their work and he is keen to promote this philosophy.
A keen Rotarian, he and his wife Elaine have two children.

Geoff Reynolds, A. Com. at Cairns for Region 1:
Geoff's career began in Charters Towers as an Honorary, going full time in 1967 as an officer/mechanic.
After two years at Roma as Deputy Super, Geoff was promoted to Superintendent at Injune in 1976.
A succession of career moves finally taking him to Cairns.
His Region is the State's largest, covering some of the most remote Stations like Normanton, Bamaga and Mutta-burra.
He will certainly have a full work schedule throughout his vast Region as new Stations come on line.
Geoff is an active Lion and currently Cairns Club President.

John Jacobson, A.Com. at Bundaberg for Region 4:
This Region will reap the benefit of
Service in all operational levels throughout NSW began for John in 1969 as a raw recruit at Junee and culminated in his appointment as Superintendent of the Central West Region based at Bathurst. In 1985 he was posted as Assistant Regional Superintendent (Ops) at Lismore.
John's hands-on, multi-trauma experience built up during a career of 23 years in the NSW Service which included direct involvement in the tragic Grafton and Kemsey bus crashes.
His experience of aerial ambulance activities at Lismore will help him in Region 4 which also includes an aerial ambulance service.

Barry Bryant, A.Com. at Beenleigh for Region 6:
Although Barry's career began in NSW, he has served since 1985 in the Queensland Ambulance Service.
His appointment in 1971 to Pomona was his first posting as Superintendent and then Superintendent at Maleny and finally to the large Centre of Beenleigh.
During his term there he supervised the design and construction of three new stations - Beenleigh, Park Ridge and Springwood, encouraged a number of staff to join a variety of planning task forces and committees and still found time to become significantly involved in the designing of ambulance vehicles.
Married with two children Barry will work from his previous Centre of Beenleigh.

Gerard Lawler, A. Com. at Rockhampton for Region 2:
Gerard's introduction to Ambulance work was at the Victorian Ambulance Officer

Training Centre where he completed his SO and SSO studies.
He has teaching qualifications for Clinical Instructor (Advanced Life Support) and General Training Officer. He was instrumental in developing and implementing Tasmania's Advanced Life Support Programme.
Gerard is a member in a number of professional institutions, and a former Council Member and Chairman, Tasmanian Division of the IAO.
A Founding Member of the Australian Critical Incident Stress Association he developed and implemented Tasmania's CIS Programme for all of that State's Emergency Services.
Gerard Lawler has a knowledge of re-structuring particularly in Tasmania where the ambulance moved away from the Health Department to Emergency Services.

THE HEADS OF DEPARTMENT:
Russell Linwood - Training and Development:
Former Australian Army Lt. Colonel Russell Linwood, appointed QAS Manager of Training and Development has spent his Army career in training, backing up his skills with the degrees Bachelor of Arts (Mil. Studies), Bachelor Educational Studies and Master of Science (Instrumental Systems).
He comes to the QAS from his position of Chief Instructor, Recruit Training Battalion and is the author or co-author of all the Army's "How to Train" manuals. His impressive career details will without doubt add a new dimension to the meaning of the words "training" and "development."

Dr. Gerard Fitzgerald – Medical Director, QAS., follows DR. Keith Mowatt.
A thesis on Emergency Department Triage led to a Doctor of Medicine degree from UQ in 1990 so it was not difficult at all for Gerard Fitzgerald to develop an abiding interest in the administration of Emergency Medicine Systems. A graduate in medicine in 1976, Gerard spent some years from 1979 as Registrar of the Casualty Department and became a Foundation Fellow of the Australian College for Emergency Medicine and later as Director of the Emergency Department of Ipswich Hospital.
Gerard is a Fellow of the Royal Australian College of Medical Administrators.
His work at the QAS includes developing patient care policies and protocols, supervising patient care aspects of training and research, assuring the quality and audit of patient care activities. This position has an important role of liaison with medical practitioners and other health professionals.

Robyn Pacey – Manager of Promotional Services.
Robyn has a broad background in the processes of communication and her appointment is aimed at a vital enhancement of the Service's marketing and promotional activities. As a former Chiefs-of-Staff in ABC radio news in Queensland, Robyn can also claim experience in the marketing and management of both private and public section affairs.

Along with the soon-to-be-appointed Regional PS Managers, Robyn will work to develop a range of strategies to improve all kinds of revenue levels and to upgrade the public's perception of the Service and the role of its officers.

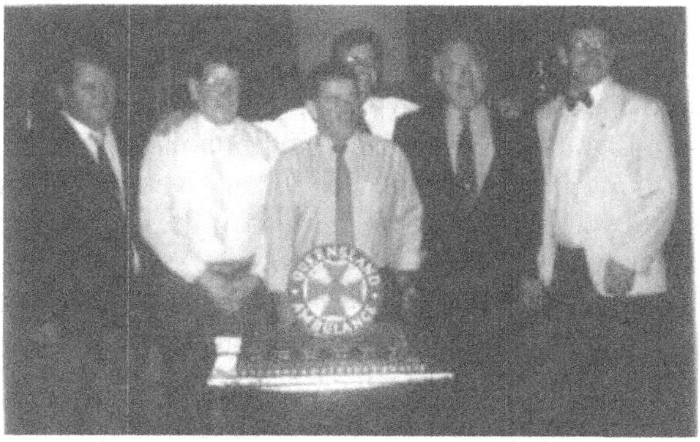

1992: the 6 Assistant Commissioners celebrate the 100 years of the Queensland Ambulance Service.

2001:
The Queensland Times article recognises the QAS: "the 110th birthday this week it is only fitting the service be remembered and applauded for their dedication and commitment to the care of others."

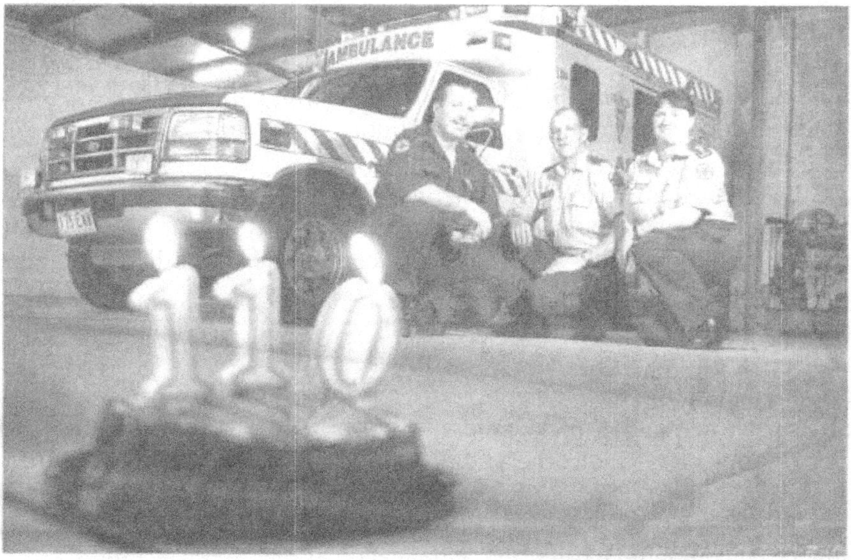

North Ipswich staff celebrate the 110 birthday of the QAS.

QAS QUALIFICATIONS INTRODUCED OVER 25 YEARS.

1991 Associate Diploma Applied Science (Ambulance) – this was the first sub tertiary program that all paramedics were required to complete to meet the minimum standard for a Paramedic in the QAS. This gave the transition to higher level programs for paramedics to where a Bachelors degree is the minimum entry requirement in QAS.

1991 Pilot scheme by QATB Ipswich for Intravenous cannulation with infusion by A/Os at scene. The start of the delivery of serious Emergency procedures

1993 Diploma Applied Science (Ambulance) = this raised the minimum educational and clinical standard for an Advanced Care Paramedic.

1995 Advanced Diploma (Intensive Care) = this was the educational and clinical standard for the Intensive Care paramedics.

After more than 20 years of working for the introduction of the administration of Advanced Life Support by certified Ambulance Officers, the Advanced Diploma in Health Science (Pre-Hospital Care) was up and running and Queensland had its first Paramedics in the field.

Intensive Care Paramedics work as a team of 2 officers - a qualified Paramedic as the Mentor, and a student Paramedic.

A CASE HISTORY of such a team in 1998 :-

Mark McDonald, ICP, with a student Paramedic officer was called to a cardiac arrest at a Bowls Club, 5 minutes away from their position.

Traffic was calm at 1730 hours this Thursday evening and there were no challenges in getting to the incident.
They were informed by the Coordination centre that Cardio Pulmonary Resuscitation was being performed at scene by lay people.
They requested a backup crew, but these would take another 5 minutes to reach them.
The action is given in the first person :-
"On arrival my partner and I picked up the defibrillator, Paramedics drug kit, bag/mask resuscitator and endotracheal intubation kit, and stepped quickly to the patient.

As we approached we could see that the patient was in the lateral position and we were informed that the patient had started to breathe.
We carried out a primary assessment ------*the patient was not breathing and did not have a pulse* -- I requested the bystander,[who had been assisting], to recommence External Chest Compressions whilst we prepared Advanced Life Support procedures.

My partner readied the cardiac monitor /defibrillator and *I intubated the patient.*

The patient's heart was in Ventricular Fibrillation and *one shock at 200 joules was administered* with no change to the patient.
Adrenaline 2 mgs was administered via the endotracheal tube and Intravenous access was achieved, ie, the patient was cannulated.

ECC and ventilations were still being carried out by the bystanders under supervision.

Shortly after the Adrenaline (combined with CPR), the *patient had a return of pulse and started to breathe*. The patients GCS improved and she started to bite down on the endotracheal tube.
The backup crew arrived.

One Officer was asked to set up some IV fluids (Hartmanns solution) and the other Officer was asked to get "us" ready for transport. This process reduces the time factor and the patient reaches definitive Medical Care in a shorter time scale. Just good, logistical, patient management practice.

As this was still a life threatening medical emergency it was imperative the patient stayed intubated so that optimum airway management could be achieved.

I elected to sedate the patient and after taking basic vital signs especially the patient s blood pressure, a mixture of Morphine and Midazolam was titrated to sedate the patient.

This was repeated approximately 15 minutes later whilst enroute to the hospital.

During transport the senior Medical Officer in the emergency department was contacted and was informed of what had occurred, treatment initiated, and current state of the patient - an ETA to the hospital was given.

On arrival at the hospital the staff were waiting in the resuscitation room.
We gave a handover report and then wrote up our Ambulance Report form.

We cleaned and restocked the Unit and were ready for another client.

We visited the patient two days later in the Critical Care Department. The patient was sitting up out of bed, talking, but had no memory of the event whatsoever."

Yes, the delivery of Pre-hospital Emergency Care by the Ambulance Service in Queensland had truly arrived.

FURTHER QAS QUALIFICATIONS INTRODUCED OVER THE 25 YEARS.

2000	Qld University Technology introduced a Bachelor's Degree.
2012	QAS now graduate entry to be a paramedic is a Bachelor's Degree
2012	**7 Regions change to 15 Local Ambulance service Networks:** this aligned the QAS with Q Health Services Networks to ensure better alignment of patient flow and care.
2015	Intensive Care Paramedics now designated as Critical Care Paramedics. CCP in the QAS requires a graduate Diploma or Masters qualification.

THE QAS – 2013 Case history:

The introduction of intravenous cannulation and Coronary Care in 1986 at QATB Ipswich returns priceless procedures in 2013 for a retiree.

At 10.38am the lady was not feeling well and quietly called her husband.

He asked the right questions and professionally observed that his wife presented as a typical heart attack – 1. Cold, clammy skin on her forehead 2. Nausea 3. Heavy weight on chest – that was enough - he immediately rang 000.

An Ambulance crew of three Paramedics arrived:-
Student AO asked from listed questions and recorded observations as per QAS Procedures and Protocols - aspirin immediately and IV cannulation inserted.

Paramedic attached ECG leads and ran off a 12 lead ECG advising the ICP.

The Intensive Care Paramedic supervised drug therapy of Glyceryl Trinitrate a vasodilator, Ondansetron for nausea, and Morphine for pain relief.
(QAS procedures and IC Paramedics are recognised as of world standard.)

The local Emergency Department was contacted whilst the patient was stretchered into the Ambulance and transported to the local Hospital.
Immediate tests, a 12 lead ECG and infusion set up with drug therapy continued – the Cardiologist advised immediate transfer to Prince Charles I.C.U.

Transported by Ambulance crew with Senior Nurse accompanying the patient under lights and siren to Prince Charles Hospital.

After assessment at CCU the patient was taken for an Angiograph which showed stenosis of four ventricular arteries of 100%, 90%, 70%, and 60%.
Stents were successfully inserted into the three worst.

The patient was returned to the CCU by 6pm, the main crisis was over.

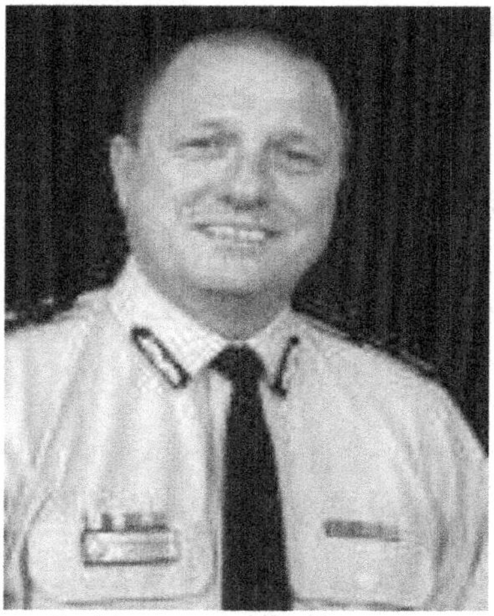

2016 – Commissioner Queensland Ambulance Service:

QAS Commissioner, Russell Bowles, ASM

Russell Bowles began his career with the QAS in January 1981 as a cadet at Rockhampton and then Ipswich attaining the rank of qualified ambulance officer in 1983 where he gained further experience as a Paramedic and then continued at Mount Isa and the Gold Coast.

He holds a Master of Business Administration and has worked in numerous management positions including area manager for the Sunshine Coast and Assistant Commissioner for the central and Brisbane regions before being appointed Deputy Commissioner in August 2008.

As Deputy Commissioner, Russell played an important role in the implementation of recommendations from the QAS Audit in 2007, which saw a renewed focus on frontline service delivery within the service and operational effectiveness.

Russell Bowles was appointed Commissioner of the Queensland Ambulance Service (QAS) in June 2011. As Commissioner, Russell has implemented a number of structural, technical and operational reforms resulting in significant service delivery improvements across a range of ambulance performance measures.

APPENDIX

Q.A.T.B. IPSWICH IN-HOSPITAL TRAINING DOCUMENTS - 1980
Step. 1 – 3

LEGEND

EXPLAINED:	SHOWN BY DOCTOR OR REG. NURSE.
OBSERVED:	OFFICER ABLE TO NOTE SPECIFIC CONDITION OR TECHNIQUE.
SUPERVISED:	OFFICER CARRIES OUT SPECIFIC TECHNIQUE UNDER SUPERVISION.
COMPETENT:	OFFICER CARRIES OUT SPECIFIC TECHNIQUE AS DIRECTED WITHOUT ASSITANCE, UNDER OBSERVATION.
SIGNATURE:	SIGNED OFF BY DOCTOR ONLY IF ASSESSED AS COMPETENT. NO TIME LIMIT

PATIENT OBSERVATION
THEATRE: Experienced, Observed, Supervised, Completed, Signed
[columns under the above had to be initialled, dated, then signed off.]

SKIN COLOUR
NORMAL
SHOCK
BLOOD LOSS
PULSE
NORMAL
SHOCK
CHEST MOVEMENT
NORMAL
POSITIVE PRESSURE
INFLATION ONE LUNG ONLY
BREATH SOUND (STETH.)

INFLATION BOTH LUNGS

THEATRE AIRWAY MANAGEMENT

ESTABLISH IF BREATHING:
AIR MOVEMENT (CUPPED HAND)
CHEST MOVEMENT
DIAPHRAGM MOVEMENT

ESTABLISH IF OBSTRUCTED:
AIR MOVEMENT
CHEST MOVEMENT
DIAPHRAGM MOVEMENT
ACTUAL VENTILATION
COMPARE BREATHING ATTEMPTS
TO ACTUAL VENTILATION

PATIENT AIRWAY
HEAD TILT
JAW SUPPORT
ART. AIRWAY
LATERAL POSITON
MONITOR BREATHS

NON BREATHING

BAG & MASK

CORRECT HEAD POSITION
CORRECT MASK POSITION
GOOD SEAL
GOOD JAW SUPPORT
CORRECT INFLATION PRESSURE.
RECOG. VENTILATION
RECOG. OBSTRUCTED AIRWAY
ABILITY TO CORRECT
NO STOMACH INFLATION
CORRECT THE ABOVE

VISUALISED VOCAL COURDS.
KNOWN LANDMARKS

ASPIRATED PATIENT

THEATRE

INFLUSION
LIST & INFUSIONS
KNOW WHY THEY ARE USED
SET UP A GIVING SET
OPTIMUM HEIGHT
CONTRA INDICATIONS
EMERGENCY NEEDLE SIZE
COLOUR CODE FOR NEEDLES
WHAT VEINS TO CHOOSE
WHERE TO START 1ST
EMERGENCY USNI PUNCTURE
ASEPTIC TECHNIQUE
AFIXING NEEDLE TO ARM

INSERTING BUTTERFLY

INSERTING CANNULAS

SETTING UP FOR INTUBATION

RECOVERY

PULSE
RADIAL
CAROTID
DORSALES PEDUE
DIFFERING TYPES & PULSE

B/P
APPLY ACUFF
DETERMINE B/P
1 PATPATION
2 AUSCULTATION
RECORD B/P
DENOTE LOW B/P
GIVE POSSIBLE REASONS

RECOVERY
STATE OF CONSCIOUSNESS

COLOUR

IPSWICH EMEGENCY CARE SYSTEM

Any Pre-hospital Care system has to be a harmonious co-operation between all members of the Health Care team.

On my appointment to Q.A.T.B. Ipswich Centre in November of 1979 I set objectives and developed strategies to provide Emergency treatment and Pre-hospital care to National standards within five years for the Ipswich community.

This was introduced in steps by educating and training staff to each level, so that they were capable and willing to advance to the next step.

If I had declared my full plan of the future Service it would not have succeeded because some officers would have been totally negative, and some intimidated, a few would have been enthusiastic, but *all would have been lost through Industrial procrastination of wanting reward before ability to provide.*

[later in the program one of my potentially top officers remarked, " but what if the Super goes, what will happen then ?"
He of course did not know that a good administrator has everything documented, and each step set in concrete, so that even if he moved, then it would be more than difficult to change anything.]

Step 1. Staff training to improve skills, education to give understanding and reasoning for the administration of treatments and procedures. (Dec.79.)
Public education in resuscitation and First aid to assist in primary care.

This was achieved by :-
(1) group lectures and individual tuition.
(2) increased intake to the State Training School.
(3) liaise with Dr. T. Mulhearn the medical Superintendent of Ipswich Regional Hospital and with Dr. S. Bedford specialist anaesthetist in regard to in-hospital training in Theatre and Recovery, after a base level of knowledge and skills was achieved by the officer. (Jan. 80.) app.ix.
NB.: This also established communication between Ambulance and Hospital staff - they now spoke in the same language.
(4) Talks to public groups and weekly classes in First aid, which provided assistance in Primary patient care.

Step 2. Provision of adequate Finance.
To finance the expected increase in staff, the provision of training aids, update of equipment and vehicles, the subscription rate was increased and Service clubs approached for support. This was not opposed by the community as they were receiving value for money.

Step 3. Upgrading of Equipment.
The actual upgrading of Equipment was through the provision of training aids for Resuscitation/ Cardiac procedures/infusion and textbooks, infant air vivas [resuscitators], suction units, collapsible trolley stretchers, and the first air-conditioned Special Care Ambulance unit.
Step 4. Selection process for the appointment of Honorary officers.

The provision for future staff had to be planned at this stage, because with the conviction that pass/fail had to be the requisite of future Training School courses, it was the responsibility of the Committee to select future officers on their ability to pass such courses and on their potential as future officers.

Step 5. The provision of suitable Ambulance Units.

The Modular Emergency Ambulance Unit was provided as it had room to move and work, ample but not excessive storage space. I carried out some renovations for the efficient arrangement of equipment and added access door on the off road side of the Unit.

Officers cannot work efficiently nor effectively if the working area is restrictive or has projecting storage compartments.

To adequately treat a serious trauma case or an arrest by resuscitation it may be necessary to have a minimum of three people working in the rear compartment.

The first Modular Ambulance Unit in April 82, from a Lion's Club donation which provided space for officers to administer good patient care -two officer crews by May 82.- four Modular units in 1985- and six by 1986, each with identical shelves and cupboards, with the same equipment and gear stored in the same places in each vehicle.

Step 6. Upgrading of skills.

After staff training had progressed to this point where all staff had attained competency in all basic life support skills the In-hospital training was upgraded in Theatre to assisting in Intubation and cannulation and to progress through the Emergency Department for all Senior Officers and potential Senior Officers.

Following Stage 2 and 3 Training School notes, but with a set procedure for documenting practical assessments, officers were trained in establishing and maintaining an I.V. line, airway management and ventilation - certification was reached by 1983.

Step 7. The Appointment of Senior Ambulance Officers.

The criteria for the appointment of senior Ambulance officers on their demonstrated knowledge and skills was established at Ipswich, and the five Senior Officers were appointed in August 1983.

[this was not achieved without some Union intervention as this was the first time officers had to *pass* tests to qualify; but all their claims were unsuccessful because I had given all officers equal training, and carried out all tests in a fair and equitable manner, using qualified and neutral examiners.]

Step 8. Maintenance of Skills - further upgrade in training.

The need for the supervision of procedures and the maintenance of Standards was addressed by the appointment of a Station Officer with the responsibility for staff training and the maintenance of Standards of treatments. Nov. 1983.

Officers were now provided with training programmes and exposed to training situations which were to provide them with an 'appreciation' of the patients injuries and overall condition in relation to the situation and time frame.
eg. type of injury, stable or deteriorating; time factor; on-site resuscitation or definitive Medical care ?

It was and is my belief that the 'appreciation' of the patient's condition is one of the most important aspects in Pre-hospital care - for this will dictate all initiatives, treatments and actions, which will directly effect the patients level of recovery, and their return to a quality of life.

Retrospective analysis of Patient-care Report forms was introduced.

Step 9. Communications and Procedures.

Now that a high standard of Patient care was being provided, and equipment and vehicles had been updated, the next need was for Communication procedures and Emergency procedures.

I developed an Operational Multiple Casualty Management Plan with procedures for the management of emergency situations in an escalating pattern from one patient or casualty to a Major Emergency of up to thirty patients, and then to the Disaster arrangements.

Portable 2-way radios; Tara radio/ telephone bridgeing system and a Beeper calling systems for Senior officers and Medical officers on-call, were all co-ordinated in the communication procedures.

Step 10. The establishment of levels of Command and the Supervision of Staff.

It was now time to officially establish Emergency crews of two officers, one being a Senior Ambulance Officer with the responsibility to initiate pre-hospital care and to supervise treatments and procedures.

The second officer to be competent in all Basic Life Support skills.

A further five Senior Officers were appointed on ability and demonstration of knowledge and skills, bringing the total to ten Senior officers on roster and two others for relief duties - this by August 1984.

The appointment on ability was not only necessary for the standard of care but it was essential that the Senior officer had recognised certification of his knowledge and skills for his authority as the Senior crew member and also for Medico-legal support in relation to specialised skills.

Step 11. The Final Phase.

1 - A percentage of the Public now trained in basic resuscitation.
2 - training and staff support established.
3 - Operational procedures tabulated and published.
4 - Emergency units and equipment to a high standard.
5 - Communications in place.
6 - Reporting procedures and retrospective analysis of emergency cases.
7 - Emergency units crewed by a Senior Officer and a second officer.
8 - 'Back - up' crews were available.
9 - Medical Officers were on-call for Retrievals.
10 - Certified procedures for on-site cannulation and infusion was in place and administered to designated casualties.

This established Pre - hospital care system was in place and tested by 1986 when pre-hospital Coronary care was introduced.

Ipswich Centre Committee was thus able to provide a service to National standards, demonstrated not only by the competence of the officers but more importantly by achieving excellence in Patient-care under all conditions.

When I went to Ipswich I had encouraged officers to attend training lectures and educational seminars and conferences to increase their knowledge of current techniques and to gain an understanding of why certain treatments are administered and how the body reacts to illness and trauma.

At the same time I would remind officers of their responsibility to administer correct treatments, and to be sure of the authority of such treatments, eg. :-
whenever they attended any lecture or talk, [even by me], they should concentrate

with an open mind on what was being said so as not to miss any information, to ask questions and to take notes if necessary, BUT, *they should then examine :-*

1. The speakers credentials and authority.
2. The speakers track record - if they had ever actually worked in the field with results
3. To then refer to the respective text book or document and check on the subject.

If all this supported what was said and claimed - then use it with authority.

My aim was to gain a core of well informed officers who were confident in their knowledge because they only used accredited treatments which they had checked and researched; this also initiated a regime of self study.

The Standard of this total System was proven on two fronts:

(1) The report by Potter and Goldstein on Pre-hospital Intensive Care and Standard Ambulance Systems in Trauma Cases investigated from late 1984 and published in 1986, lists one case attended by an Ipswich Unit with two officer crew, as being the patient with the highest ISS score with which survival occurred, (a patient with extensive injuries) - a standard above all other States in the research survey.

(2) Coronary Care documented records of cases which includes the percentage of 'saves' from cardiac arrest patients who were defibrillated and later discharged from hospital - this as high as 16 %.
The Ipswich Centre was providing patient care of a high standard with advanced techniques, therefore to ensure protection for all, communications were updated with the installation of sophisticated Voice Logging equipment which recorded all telephone and radio calls in and out of the Centre.
This not only allowed for retrospective analysis but it provided an instant recall facility which gave the Controllers greater security and support.

Note:- Documentation relating to monitoring and defibrillation of patients in cardiac arrest with ventricular fibrillation or ventricular tachycardia, using Life Pac manual machines is shown in appendix ix.

To take an idea and make it happen takes a great deal of commitment, and this relates to time and effort - you think and breathe every step of the project, everything that you do, everything that occurs on the job and at public functions has a bearing on the current and final success or not of the project; you must be forever vigilant to nurse and except every assistance; to recognise and encourage effort, but also to identify any inefficiency or slackness with the appropriate corrective comment and action.
At times the lazy or inefficient or outright 'whinger' made things difficult with their

repeated negative and defeatist comments and complaints, which were often brought to me by the Union rep, because, " I represent the staff and speak on their behalf," as he would say, to which I would reply, "no, you are only representing 3 % of the staff, 3 out of 60, if that."

The main problem was that if the staff knew what training and changes I had planned for them and the service over the five years, they would have been 'scared stiff' and would have been totally uncooperative, but taking things step by step allowed them to progress with knowledge and with security.

But these defeatist attitudes, especially if one of the better type of officer fell for the 'bullet makers' tripe, sometimes made me feel, 'why keep on, why sacrifice your own time to lift their status and conditions, why bother,' so that I had to consciously 'talk' firmly to myself, eg.- "stick to your plans, kept on the path, you know what's best, lead them through" - it got very lonely sometimes.

If you are doing to succeed you must believe in yourself and in the project/cause, and never deviate.

IPSWICH CALL CENTRE:

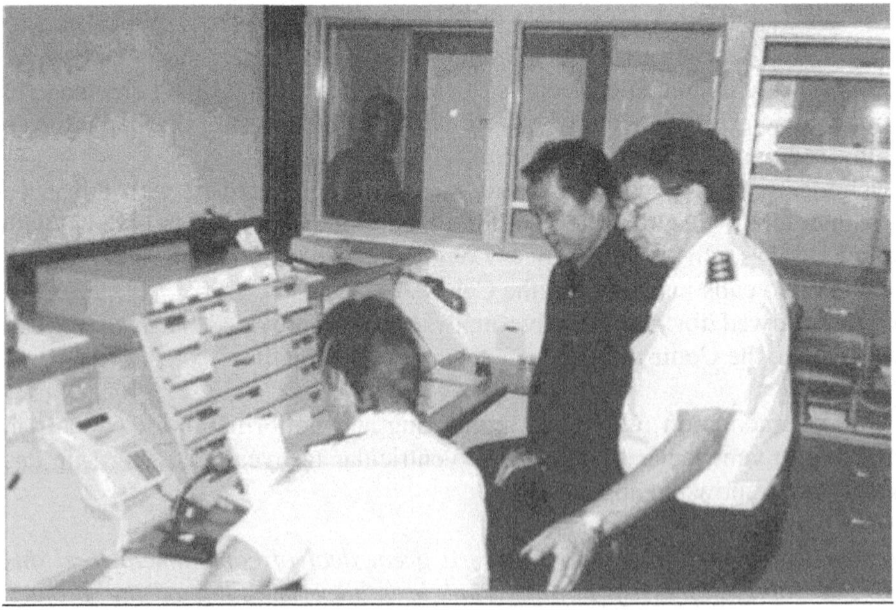

Superintendent demonstrates the functions of the Ipswich Call Centre to Major William Sng from National University Hospital Singapore.

Places for 4 Station Officers at L shaped desk
Emergency lines with specific ring tone.

Inquiry line with normal tone - 4 lines available.
Direct line to/from IGH Emergency Department.
Bridgeing phone with Unit 2 way radio to Director.
2 phone lines for Office to be used in emergencies for outgoing calls only.

Call sheets (removed with other items to maintain confidentiality for photo) in slots in front of Officer coded according to their grade. These are clipped with Report form on completion on return to Centre. This becomes the source document for Retrospective analysis and for Administration records.

1.5.1985 – the following EXTRACT continues from the previous paper presented at the Gold Coast Education Centre, on "The Development of the Combined Ambulance/Medical Pre-hospital Care System for Ipswich" by Supt. M.C. McDonald, introduced by Dr. Phil Kay, Director Gold Coast Hospital, Accident and Emergency Department.

EXTRACTS TAKEN FROM PRESENTATION PAPERS :

1. **PRIMARY ASSESSMENT AT THE ACCIDENT SCENE – BLS or ALS or WHAT?**
2. **INFUSION AT SCENE.**
3. **MEDICAL TEAMS AT SCENE**

(OH) Primary assessment procedure. 34

The Officer notifies control etc. etc.

(OH) On this primary assessment the A/O decides—

(SLIDE) Patient with life threatening condition.

If it is obvious that the patient is suffering from a life threatening condition - then Control is alerted with the report "car 4 to Control, have patient with life threatening condition - transporting as soon as possible - will request hospital link later - out". The Officers will carry out minimum B.L.S. AIRWAY, HAEMORRHAGE CONTROL, CERVICAL COLLAR, TEMPORARY IMMOBILISATION, LOAD, VITAL SIGNS AND TRANSPORTS.

On transporting the Officers would link with A. & E. Senior M.O. and give the following information.

(OH) Radio report - Ambulance Officer to Senior Medical Officer standard report

Further information can be given from the accident report form - as now recommended by the South Eastern Zone.

(OH) Report form overdoes. (explain from report form).

The other situation for early transport is the situation may change and the patient who presents with altered state of consciousness.

*(SLIDE) Riverview Smash-sub dural.

May deteriate - in this case a 21 year old male unconscious, compound # left tib and fib and # right femur, was being rescued from entrapment by the legs.

*(SLIDE) Unequal pupils.

The patient deteriated - became increasingly restless with cries from acute pain - Senior STaff Officer diagnosed sub dural haemotoma with inter-crannial pressure, he stopped the rescues and forcibly extricated the victims legs and transported as soon as possible.

THIS ACTION IS SUPPORTED BY RESEARCH.

In the Boston study patients with trauma score of 1 - 3 have massive physiologic derangement and a high predicted mortality and therefore require rapid transportation and immediate surgery, notwithstanding this statement, the term 'scoop and run' is an exaggeration, because some basic life support MUST be carried out, cervical collar, airway management, suction, immobilisation (temporary if needed) etc. as the Boston Study also states:-

However, time is also required for BLS care. This includes the time it takes to determine the vital signs, secure the patient to the stretcher in such a way as to protect against further spinal or long bone injur, move from the scene of injury into the Ambulance, and travel to the Hospital.

Donald D. Trunkey says - "In the critically injured patient the goal should be to reduce the time from injury to definitive surgical care, and yet provide resuscitation that will increase the chances of the patient arriving 'alive' at the Hospital".

The other side of transporting early is the so called "quick trip" or "scoop and run."

(SLIDE) Night shot if available - transporting.

The rapid trip to Hospital is also a misconception. The Ambulance has to reach the Hospital, with all on Board, in one piece - also the Officers working on the patient must be able to work effectively - notwithstanding that kynetic and centrifugal forces in a speeding Ambulance, subject the patient to these forces also, and thus change inter-crannial pressure and increase haemorrhage etc. etc. etc.

All of us have worked in the back of an Ambulance.

(SLIDE) Smash - Coal truck and Doctor.

If the Ambulance Officer requires a Doctor he must justify this by: Primary assessment of situation and patient.

(1) Injury and entrapment = time delay.

(2) Serious injury, (as per procedure list) + distance and/or road traffic conditions = time delay.

(3) Multipe casualties with multiple injuries = time delay before transport.

After initiating medical assistance the Senior Ambulance Officer then returns to the immediate scene, and with his crewman continues with B.L.S. and secondary assessment. This includes vital signs and full patient examination.

(SLIDE) Tarampa roadside smash.

(OH) Accident report form M.V.A. multipe fractures etc. (explain information on sheet)

The Ipswich system has developed towards establishing pre-hospital care (in the life threatening and medical trauma range) under direct Medical supervision.

(SLIDE) Arrival at Hospital - Beasley.

Our own experience has shown the benefits to the patient who receives infusion or intubation etc. - and overseas research back this up.

Mannix says full BLS plus infusion, if any signs of hypovolaemia.

Jacobs and Berrizbeitia say, full BLS plus infusion, if it will not delay transport.

Trunkey says establishing an IV line takes time, so that an assessment must be made between, time taken to start an IV volume-push possible, and transport time.

An Ambulance Officer should initiate oxygen therapy before his patient presents as hypoxic, for he should diagnose and appreciate the patients condition and the inevitable deteriation.

In the same sense the Senior Ambulance Officer should appreciate the patient suffering blood loss in his primary assessment and should link with the Senior M.O. at A. & E. to ascertain the appropriate procedure.

(SLIDES) AMBULANCE OFFICER IN UNIT - CONTROL/A. & E.

In this mid trauma range (as in all emergencies) we have a back-up system where A/O's at scene can request Senior personnel back-up, or A/O back-up - what ever - and they will get it - I've attended many times, when the back-up crew worked with the attending 2 man crew giving ALS at the same time as BLS there was no time extension - this is supported by Boston Trauma Study.

Our data showed that in the urban Boston setting, an average of 31 minutes was required to clinically evaluate patients, prepare for transport, and drive to a Hospital. The pre-hospital treatment time was somewhat shorter (25 minutes on average) for patients with more severe trauma (TS 1-3). ALS interventions carried out in synchrony with BLS care, did not require any significant additional time.

Analysis of the results shows that ALS intervention caused an improvement in the immediate physiologic status of serious trauma patients. The TS of patients treated by paramedics increased significantly en route to the Hospital, and that of BLS patients remained unchanged. This finding is not surprising; the beneficial hemodynamic effects of pneumatic anti-shock garments and intravenous crystalloids are well documented (5,16) in documented cases at Ipswich compared to the Boston study.

Information from the journal of trauma vol. 24-1 from the Boston emergency study, give BLS at scene plus transport to Hospital as an averaage of 31 minutes + response - vol. 23-6 on pattens in management of motor vehicle accident victims gives the average infield plus transport time as 37 minutes + response time - when examining the time factor, response time must always be considered. I.E. time from injury to arrival at scene.

In documented M.V.A. cases at Ipswich compared to the Boston Study, the average time for Ipswich from response, to pre-hospital care,to transport to Hospital to arrival at Hospital as 50 minutes. (min. case 7 mins.) - response 40 - 45.

(SLIDE) Unloading at Hospital, 2nd Beasley.

(SLIDE) Tractor on side.

In this category where there may be only one injured casualty, who is not trapped, and the Officers primary assessment gives no present indication of a life threatening condition.

NOTE: I said 'no present indication', reassessment of the patient must be made at regular intervals.

(SLIDE) Outside unit.

The Senior Ambulance Officer will report, no assistance required, first assessment, # femur and lacerations, patient conscious.

The Ambulance Officers would then continue with full BLS treatment.

(OH) Full procedure.

Control of haemorrhage, pain relief and immobilisation of fractures

(SLIDE) Load into Ambulance.

THEN: Secondary assessment, full patient examination at this point treatment will be changed if necessary, that is if there is evidence of blood loss from the femur, oxygen therapy will be initiated and a link with the A. & E. at I.G.H. would be requested.

The Ambulance Officer would give his report to the Senior M.O. with estimated time of arrival.

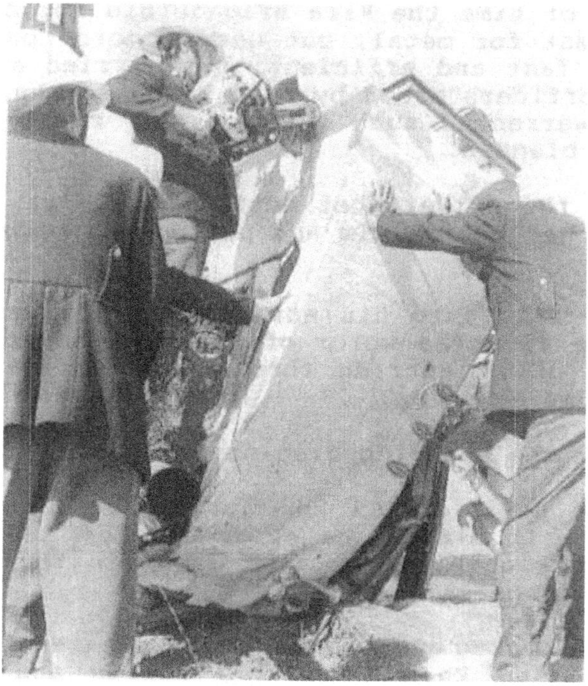

Coal transporter overturns – injured driver trapped.

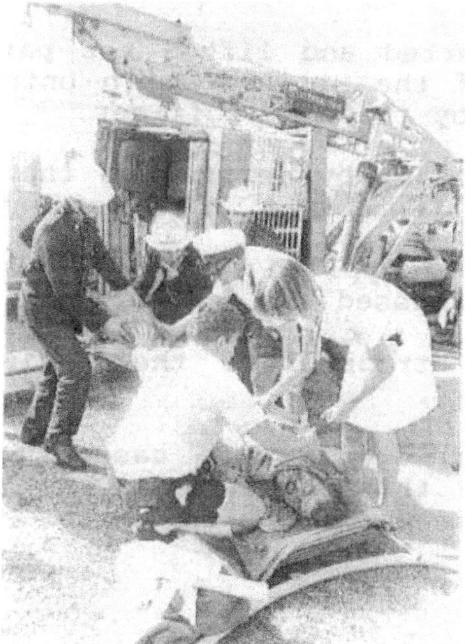

FROM THIS SYSTEM CASUALTIES ARE ARRIVING AT A. & E. IN A MUCH BETTER CONDITION.

Emergency Medicene Vol. 1, gives the criteria for Pre-Hospital care and the advantage to the patient of infusion.

Vital signs - thorough examination - basic A, B, C - oxygen - ventilation - infusion - immobilisation - hospital alerted.

I have also been asked to comment on assistance from Medical Officers at scene.

One cannot generalise so I give certain actual situations.

The fully trained Senior Doctor who has worked for the past 10 years in a totally administrative position: on the whole these Doctors if they stop, know that they are out of touch with emergency procedures and if the Ambulance crew are showing competence and give certification and request permission to put up a drip - then these Doctors are only to happy to sign the emergency report forms.

The very young and inexperienced medical intern: they will stop to assist but generally feel their inexperience, and are not willing to give permission for anything - unless they are from the same Hospital where the Ambulance Officers receive training, then permission will be given - sometimes the very young M.O., due to his own peronsal stress from feeling of inadequacy, and the belief that he should know etc., will give direct instruction to Ambulance Officers albeit inappropriate - Ambulance Officers should assist these Medical Officers.

(SLIDE) Food van.

The active G.P. who stops: He still has memories of casualty and what he did, but he has been away from the total emergency situation for so long, that when he is confronted with smashed metal, bad light, noise of traffic, with Police and Fire Brigade sirens in the distance - the disarray of the scene - the twisted body with obvious blood everywhere, just everywhere! - then he cannot be blamed if he starts to interrupt Officers in their assessments and treatments, and can only talk about getting the patient out and away (away from sight), to Medical aid and definitive care - "I have told you to move! transport that patient quickly!" - He will not give the Ambulance Officer a chance to get into any set method or procedure in his extrication or Pre-Hospital care - this Medical Officer is in every way a hindrance and a negative force, yet he is the one who complains to higher Medical Authority.

The Hospital Ward Doctor who stops: then the Intensive Care Sister from another Hospital who stops to assist: the Doctor decides to intubate and the Sister assists, BUT its beside the road and cricoid pressure is forgotten even though the Superintendent mentioned this, intubation is abandoned and the doctor and Sister take over C.P.R. - the patient is loaded and transported - the Ambulance Officer arranges for an Ambulance Officer to be at roadside to get in and assist with C.P.R. - Doctor says, don't stop! and drive past Ambulance Officer - etc.

The other G.P. who stops: says he has been away from the game for awhile but can he assist? This Doctor can be of great assistance and reassurance for the Ambulance Officer - He will either administer requred drugs, cannulate or permit the Ambulance Officer to cannulate and put up the infusion, he may even intubate if this is necessary and he is confident in his expertise - or he will quietly supervise and give his approval to the actions of the Ambulance crew.

(SLIDE) The best Medical aid is from that Centres base Hospital, because:

(AT A. & E.)

1. Communications are established.

2. The Doctor knows the Ambulance Staff.

3. Procedures have been written to give a time saving smooth flow of assistance.

4. The patient will receive the highest standard of pre-hospital care available, to whatever level is required.

The assistance from Hospital must be in the form of Senior A. & E. Doctors who know where they and everyone else are at.

(SLIDE) In A. & E.

The young Doctor who is seconded because he was the only poor bugger handy - is as lost as the inexperienced Ambulance Officer, both are willing but, what to do??

The same with assistance from Hospitals where too often different, replacement or changed staff are on duty, and these R.N. 's have no idea of the Pre-Hospital emergency situation.

Refer. Gailes Railway accident.

The following Accident Report Form refers to the case OH7 on p. 244

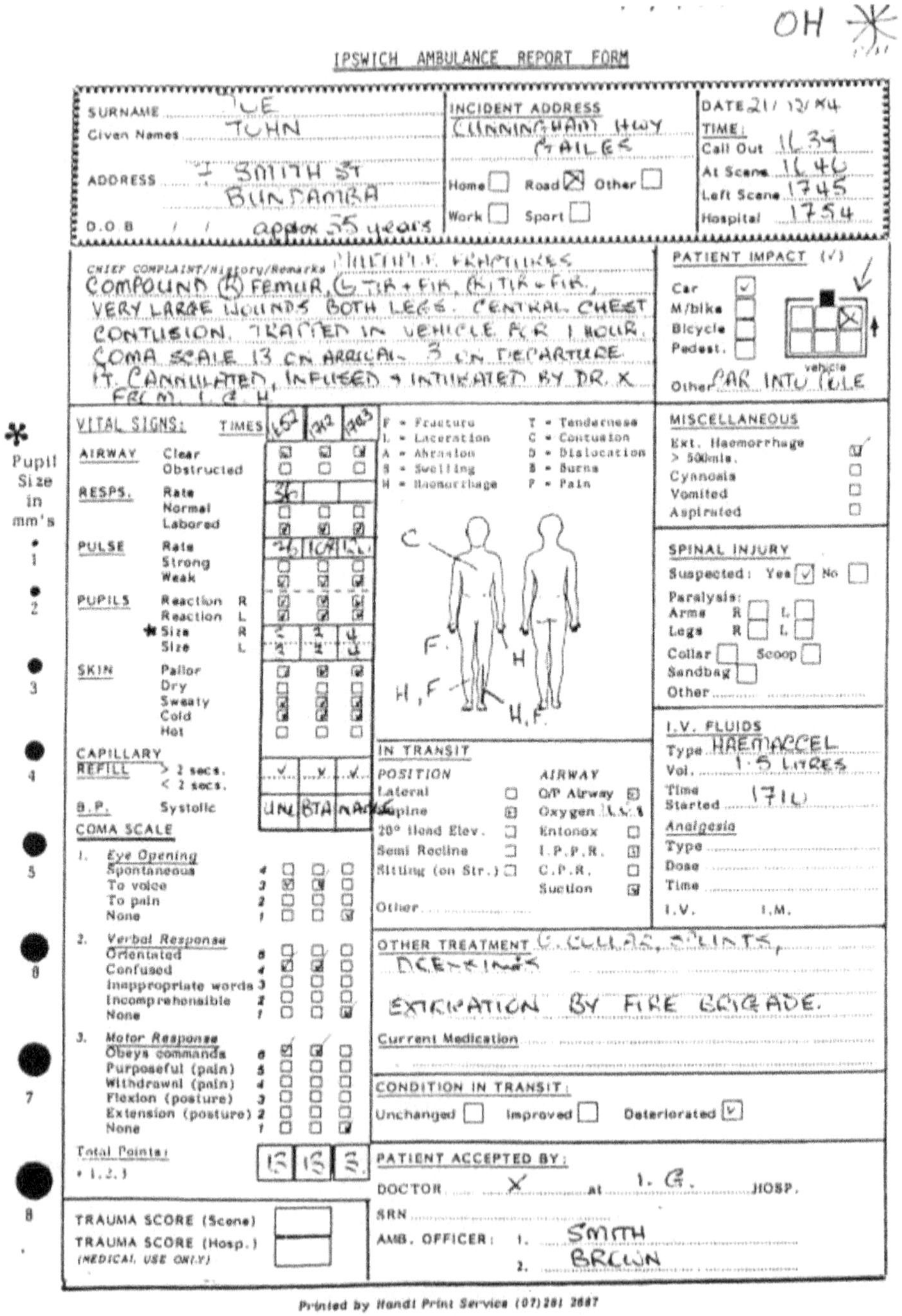

OH *

IPSWICH AMBULANCE REPORT FORM

SURNAME: LE Given Names: JOHN ADDRESS: 1 SMITH ST BUNDAMBA D.O.B. / / approx 35 years	INCIDENT ADDRESS: CUNNINGHAM HWY GAILES Home ☐ Road ☒ Other ☐ Work ☐ Sport ☐
DATE 21/12/84 TIME: Call Out 1639, At Scene 1646, Left Scene 1745, Hospital 1754	

CHIEF COMPLAINT/History/Remarks: MULTIPLE FRACTURES COMPOUND (R) FEMUR, (L) TIB + FIB, (R) TIB + FIB, VERY LARGE WOUNDS BOTH LEGS. CENTRAL CHEST CONTUSION. TRAPPED IN VEHICLE FOR 1 HOUR. COMA SCALE 13 ON ARRIVAL 3 ON DEPARTURE. PT. CANNULATED, INFUSED + INTUBATED BY DR. X FRCM, I.G.H.

PATIENT IMPACT (✓): Car ☑ M/bike ☐ Bicycle ☐ Pedest. ☐ Other CAR INTO POLE (vehicle)

VITAL SIGNS: TIMES 1652, 1712, 1723
AIRWAY Clear / Obstructed; RESPS. Rate 36, Normal, Labored; PULSE Rate 76, 108, 120, Strong, Weak; PUPILS Reaction R, Reaction L, * Size R, Size L; SKIN Pallor, Dry, Sweaty, Cold, Hot; CAPILLARY REFILL > 2 secs. < 2 secs.; B.P. Systolic UNR, BTA, NAD; COMA SCALE: 1. Eye Opening (Spontaneous 4, To voice 3, To pain 2, None 1); 2. Verbal Response (Orientated 5, Confused 4, Inappropriate words 3, Incomprehensible 2, None 1); 3. Motor Response (Obeys commands 6, Purposeful (pain) 5, Withdrawal (pain) 4, Flexion (posture) 3, Extension (posture) 2, None 1); Total Points: 13, 13, 3 (* 1, 2, 3)

* Pupil Size in mm's: 1, 2, 3, 4, 5, 6, 7, 8

F = Fracture, L = Laceration, A = Abrasion, S = Swelling, H = Haemorrhage, T = Tenderness, C = Contusion, D = Dislocation, B = Burns, P = Pain
C, F, H, H,F, H,F

MISCELLANEOUS: Ext. Haemorrhage > 500mls. ☑ Cyanosis ☐ Vomited ☐ Aspirated ☐

SPINAL INJURY: Suspected: Yes ☑ No ☐ Paralysis: Arms R ☐ L ☐ Legs R ☐ L ☐ Collar ☐ Scoop ☐ Sandbag ☐ Other

IN TRANSIT: POSITION Lateral ☐ Supine ☒ 20° Head Elev. ☐ Semi Recline ☐ Sitting (on Str.) ☐ Other; AIRWAY O/P Airway ☒ Oxygen ☒ Entonox ☐ I.P.P.R. ☒ C.P.R. ☐ Suction ☒

I.V. FLUIDS: Type HAEMACCEL Vol. 1.5 LITRES Time Started 1716; Analgesia Type, Dose, Time, I.V. I.M.

OTHER TREATMENT: C. COLLAR, SPLINTS, DRESSINGS. EXTRICATION BY FIRE BRIGADE.
Current Medication

CONDITION IN TRANSIT: Unchanged ☐ Improved ☐ Deteriorated ☑

PATIENT ACCEPTED BY: DOCTOR X at I.G. HOSP. SRN
AMB. OFFICER: 1. SMITH 2. BROWN

TRAUMA SCORE (Scene)
TRAUMA SCORE (Hosp.) (MEDICAL USE ONLY)

Printed by Handi Print Service (07) 281 2887

The Accident Report Form introduced at Gatton and developed at Ipswich to provide a formal record of the patients signs, symptoms and injuries, but most importantly to provide a 'check list' which prompted secondary assessment.
Trauma cases which required back-up from A&E Medical Officers:

·7.

I will quickly run through some cases where Officers have called for the A. & E. Medical Officer to attend.

It can be noted that it was the Senior Medical Officer who attended in these cases, bar one.

SLIDE OF SCENE CASE 1

IDE The first case involved a 52 year old male, on 22nd August, 1980, he had a gas cylinder explode beside him, he suffered multiple fractures on the Left side from hip to foot with extensive tissue damage.

On arrival the Ambulance Officers diagnosed hypovolemic shock and also assessed that further movement would have aggravated the blood loss. They called for Doctor at scene. I collected the Senior A. & E. Medical Officer, and on arrival I assisted him to put up infusions into both arms, these were run wide open with pressure to the bags. The A/Officer continued with haemorrhage control and splinting.

After loading the patient but prior to transporting both bags of haemaccel were replaced, the Hospital was notified. In our opinion this action saved this casualties life. Mines Rescue Station

****

17 ACCIDENT REPORT FORM

Case 2 involved 2 casualties who were struck by a train at Gailes Railway Station on 22nd March, 1984.

The first Officers on primary assessment called for a Doctor and back up. A second emergency crew was dispatched and I picked up the Senior A. & E. Medical Officer.

At scene the 2 Officers carried out B.L.S. and on arrival of Doctor the patients were reassessed, then loaded immediately into separate Ambulances. The patient with a fractured femur, severe lacerations, was infused with haemaccel by an accredited Ambulance Officer and then transported.//

Doctor G. F. Gr. (who well remain nameless) intubated the critical patient J.H. with (Supt McDonald) assisting, whilst another Ambulance Officer inserted an IV line and set up a Haemaccel infusion; a third Ambulance Officer was assisting all. On Doctors instruction the 3rd R w. Officer inserted Sod. Bi-carb into the IV line. P.A.H. was informed of the patients condition and E.T.A. The patient was transported to P.A.H. and on arrival was stable, without the retrieval action taken he would have definitely been D.O.A.

****

ES

SLIDES BEASLEY

In the case the Officers at scene called for Medical assistance, and an A. & E. Medical Officer was transported to scene, but was recalled to the Hospital due to patient work load. at the Hospital (by Hosp Med. S

(OH) 8.

The Senior Ambulance Officer at the scene used the Tara link to call for a Senior Medical Officer on call and back-up.

(2 SLIDES, L. EDWARDS)

The Senior Medical Officer on call attended and infused and intubated the patient using Ambulance Officers assistance

* * * * * * *

(SLIDE) Doctor Taylor and Tracheostomy patient.

In this case the patient had a problem with his tracheostomy and the trackie cuff had ruptured, the Ambulance Officer on the case called for advice by way of 2 way link, the Senior A. & E. Medical Officer attended with back-up (satisfactory result). The patient was disconnected from the bird respirator and ventilated until the trackie tube was replaced in A. & E.

* * * * * * *

SLIDE M.V.A. AND ACCIDENT REPORT FORM. OH *

In this case the Senior Ambulance Officer of the Ambulance team, make a primary assessment, appreciated the patients critical condition and blood loss - he inserted an IV line and infused with haemaccel - called for Senior A. & E. Medical Officer to attend. On arrival this M.O. Officer confirmed Hypovoemic shock and inserted a second IV line.

This instance where the Ambulance Officer initiated the action, and the Medical Officer extended that action, demonstrates the practical application of Officer training and Medical support.

* * * * * * * *

SLIDES - (1) Scene
(2) Inserting butterfly.
(3) Outside unit.
(4) IV Line.

This case involves a collision between a semi-trailer and a truck carrying an 11 tonne scraper.

The semi overturned and the 11 tonne scraper rolled on top of the semi crushing the cabin flat. The driver was entrapped in a small area of crushed metal, and his wrist was held under pressure by part of the windscreen frame.

The Senior Ambulance Officer of the emergency crew called for back-up and Medical Officer at scene, as it was obvious it would be some time before the patient was freed.

He was monitored constantly and oxy-therapy was administered.
A butterfly was inserted to give access for drug therapy.

On being freed his compound fractured wrist was immobiled and an IV line inserte and an infusion of haemaccel commenced.

I am of the opinion that emergency Ambulance crews of accredited skills capable of carrying out emergency pre-hospital care to ALS under direct Medical command, with Senior A. & E. Medical Officers on call for direct advice and for attendance at scene if necessary, is the most efficient and cost effective approach to pre-hospital care.

SLIDE END WITH SLIDE CC - AND SATISFACTORY RESULT, THIS SLIDE TELLS IT ALL.

OFFICERS MUST PARTICIPAT : - PAPERS PRESENTED AT MEDICAL AND AMBULANCE CONFERENCES:

28.12.1975 –"A Broadening Field" IAO(Aust) at Gatton Collage, opening address by Supt. McDonald, convenor of the first Seminar in Queensland on pre-hospital emergency care – guest speakers Dr. Ian Macdonald –Infusion at scene and RN Carolyn Carlisle, who trained at PA Hospital, and is currently the first Coronary Care Instructor for MICA Officers for Victorian Ambulance Services.
4.7.1976 – "The Aims of the Institute and Seminars" IAO(Aust) Rockhampton Seminar, by M.C. McDonald
29.10.1979 – "The Assessment and Management of Roadside Casualties" Gatton Hospital presentation by Supt. McDonald.
29.6.1980 – "The Problems of Extrication and Evacuation" presented by M.C. McDonald at the Qld. Casualty Assoc. "Trauma" Seminar Ipswich Hospital.
25.1.1981- Opening address and presentation of "Rescue in the Ambulance Service" case histories, by M.C. McDonald, FIAO.
1.2.8.1981 – Rockhampton IAO(Aust.) Seminar, a supporting paper to Mrs. Carrick, "Child Abuse cases as attended by Ambulance Officers " presented by M.C. McDonald.
15-16.5.1882 – IAO(Aust) Bundaberg Workshop on Syllabus, closing address by M.C. McDonald.
12-13.11.1983- IAO(Aust) National Seminar Redlands Qld. – M.C McDonald, Chairman Qld. Div. introduced Dr. T. Livingstone, Director General of Health and Medical Services to open the Seminar followed by Dr. Noel Stevenson, FFACEM, member of the QATB SCATS and member of NEC.
30.3.1985 – Adelaide seminar, M.C. McDonald presented paper "Aspects of Extrication"
1.5.1985 – Gold Coast Education Centre, paper on "The Development of the Combined Ambulance/Medical Pre-hospital Care System for Ipswich" by Supt. M.C. McDonald, introduced by Dr. Phil Kay, Director Gold Coast Hospital, Accident and Emergency Department.
26-27.10.1985- Accident and Emergency Association weekend Conference, paper on "Medical Teams at the Accident Scene" presented by M.C. McDonald, FAIAO
9.11.1985 – IAO(Aust) AGM and Competitions Dinner – Presidents Address by Malcolm C. McDonald FAIAO, to his Excellency, Governor Tasmania, Institute Members and Distinguished Guests – which elucidated on the delivery of Pre-hospital Emergency Care and the professionalism of Ambulance Officers.

1986 Oct. 9th -10th October, as President of the IAO(Aust) Malcolm McDonald addressed the combined meeting of Ambulance Authorities in Darwin – the first Operational Officer President to address the AAA – used it to push the professionalism of A/officers and to put pressure on the QATB State Council executive members attending – expanded on the Objectives of the Institute, it's positive influence on improving Officer education, the value of Ambulance Competitions as a 'win win' for Officers, Centre and the Ambulance Authority and more.

11.10.86 Alice Springs - presenting the paper "Rescue and Retrieval" which addressed many issues – the necessity for ALS training of Officers, fluid replacement for trapped or 30 minutes from Hospital casualties; communication with Centre and Hospital. Met with Ambulance Executive officers and Institute members in the following Capital Cities:-
12.10.86 Adelaide;
14.10.86 Hobart, and finally
17.10.86 Maroochydore, - "Surfair Seminar 1986" 18-19 October, presented paper " Rescue and Retrieval"
1986 Nov. 15th- Institute AGM and National Competitions – Malcolm McDonald, FAIAO. gave the Presidents address with strong reference to the progress in the standard of Emergency Care and the professionalism of the Ambulance Officer.
1987, June 6-7- Accident and Emergency Association Conference: presentation of paper " The Ipswich Experience of Pre-hospital Coronary in Queensland" supported by response and "save" statistics, by M.C. McDonald, FIAO, AIMM, President of the Institute of Ambulance Officers (Aust.).
1987 October 17th- Opening address by M.C. McDonald at the Institute Seminar Gladstone.
1987 November 12th – M.C. McDonald, President of the Institute of Ambulance Officers (Aust.) presents his Report to the Convention of the Ambulance Authorities Australia Canberra.
1987, Nov. 13th – Outgoing Presidents address to the AGM Dinner at Ballarat, Victoria, followed by his introduction of the duly elected President from 1987, Keith Campbell.
1988, June 30th – National Seminar Ipswich "Coronary Care - Pre Hospital life Support" M.C. McDonald, PP and Chairman of the Qld. Division of IAO(Aust.), gave the Address at the Conference Banquet.
1992 - International Medical Conference – at Jupiter's Casino, Gold Coast, Conference Chairman and Convenor, QAS Assist Commissioner M.C. McDonald, ex Supt. QATB Ipswich presented the Closing Address – 477 delegates from 22 countries attended. Organising Committee members: Mick Davis, President IAO(Aust); Mike Harrison, Physio Control Corporation; Phil Honan, Phoenix Scientific Industries; Martin Kelly, Vice Chairman Qld. Div. IAO(Aust); Col Nash, QAS Training Officer.

Australian Counter Disaster College Certificates:
Hazard Analysis for Disaster managers.
Hazardous Material Management-Emergency Situations.
Disaster Response Management.
Planning for Counter Disaster Executives.
Seminar - Public Disaster Education and Public Awareness.
Practical experience :
On-site Commander- Ambulance at numerous Major Emergency situations.
Exercises – Major Disaster.
Convenor of a number of Combined Emergency Services Disaster Exercises.

THE VARIOUS ACTS and REGULATIONS:
The C.A.T.B., the City Ambulance Transport Brigade was formed in 1892, to be the first formal Ambulance Service in Queensland
In 1897 the C.A.T.B. was gazetted under the "Hospitals Act."
This unique service spread further afield with Centres established at Townsville, Charters Towers, Rockhampton, Warwick and Ipswich; some affiliated with the C.A.T.B. and some independent.
In 1902 a change in the authority of the service was required and the Q.A.T.B.H. (Queensland Ambulance Transport Brigade Hospital) was established under the Hospitals Act, allowing autonomy to each Centre Committee to operate under the amended "Rules" and a State Executive to provide co-ordination between all Committees and to allow distribution of Government subsidies.
In 1910 Rules were framed for the Q.A.T.B.H., and amended in 1919.
In 1927 the Ambulance Regulations were introduced.
In 1967 the "Ambulance Services Act of 1967" was passed by Parliament, introducing major changes to the administration of the QATB with the establishment of the 'State Council of the Queensland Ambulance Transport Brigade' with the service still responsible to the Minister for Health.
This Act was amended in 1986 with the State Council of 29 members of being replaced by **the 'Ambulance Services Board'** of 9 members - there were 96 independent QATB Committees.
The QATB Training School commenced in June 1970, with the Chief Training Officer Cliff Coddington from the NSWs Ambulance Service - the author attended Stage 1 Course 1.
AUTHORS AMBULANCE SERVICE:
Malcolm C. McDonald, Esq, OAM, FPA., joined the Queensland Ambulance Service in 1959 as an Honorary Officer at QATB Cairns, then as a permanent Officer at Julia Creek in 1962 and to Rockhampton Centre in 1964 where he also served as an Aerial Ambulance Attendant in the Central Qld. Aerial Ambulance.
Appointed Superintendent of Wowan Centre in 1969 then Maleny Centre and to Gatton Centre in 1973. Assistant Commissioner Region 5, Brisbane 1991.
A Founder Member of the Institute of Ambulance Officers (Aust.) in 1973 and Chairman of the Queensland Division.
Elected the first Operational Officer to the position of National President of the Institute in 1984.
Organised the first Pre-hospital Care Seminar in Qld at Gatton in 1975.
Appointed Superintendent of QATB Ipswich in 1979, fully operational to Coronary Care in 1986.
Developed the Pre-hospital Emergency Care system for the QATB Ipswich District.
Appointed 27.3.1991 as Convenor of the Ministerial Task force to write 'The Ambulance Service Act' and for the Manual of Operational Procedures.
Appointed Assistant Commissioner, QAS, Metropolitan Region 5 & retired in 1993.
Currently Secretariat of the Continuing Professional Development program.
Awarded the 50 year QAS service medal on 8.9.2015

BIBLIOGRAPHY.

The Australian Medical Corps-	Textbook.
A Mountain Grows from a Mole Hill – history of C.A.T.B. -	S.C.Warrian, certified by Jack, Brown & Siegman.
Manual of Splints &Appliances for the treatment of bone and joint injuries-	The British Red-Cross society 1917.
Warwick & Tunstall's First Aid to the injured and sick.	
An Advanced Ambulance Handbook.	F.C. Nichol, 1939
Minutes – C.A.T.B. meetings.	Records.
The Story of a Vital Service -	J & C Bell-Booth.
REPORT- Conference on the Training of Ambulance Officers -	Dr. J.A. McDonnell, Monash University.
History of the Queensland Ambulance Service -	J.A. Ryan
Minutes – Q.A.T.B. meetings-	Records.
Q.A.T.B. Annual Reports -	Records.
Personal Diaries and Papers -	M.C. McDonald, Supt. & A.Comm.
Queensland Newspapers -	Courier Mail & Queensland Times.
Institute of Ambulance Officers.	Documents.
Coronary Care Documentation -	D. Statham, Q.A.T.B. Ipswich.
Australian Ambulance Services-	Bain, Robertson & Jamieson.
Controlled Trial of: Pre-Hospital Intensive Care & Standard Ambulance Services -	Potter & Goldstein. 1986
Papers & Presentations 1975 – 1992-	M.C. McDonald, FIAO, AIMM.
History of the Queensland Ambulance Service -	Ernest Bradley, OAM. 1993.
The Ipswich Hospital 1860 – 1991-	Ross Patrick. 1993
TRUST ME – I'm an Ambulance Officer -	M.C. McDonald, OAM. 1993.

AUTHOR'S PROFILE.

Malcolm Cameron McDonald, Esq., OAM., O. St. J., FPA., LMPA.

Born in Cairns in 1934 and lived the free lifestyle of a youngster in the low populated, tropical, coastal area.

Educated at the Cairns High and Technical College, participating in the sports of Foot running and member of the 1st Rugby League Team.

As a teenager worked for the Qld. Railway Department and as a QRAC First Aid officer and Lecturer.
Examined and competed annually in Queensland Railway Ambulance Corps Competitions, gaining awards of "The Thallon Medal" and "The Minister for Transport Gold Medal" as well as Individual Competition events.

Played Hockey to 'A' grade standard, representing Ipswich 'Colts' and Cairns North team.

Served in the RAAF in 10 (Operational) Squadron as an Armament Fitter for National Service and on the RAAF Reserve.

Took up the sport of amateur Motorcycle Scramble racing for a couple of years.

Joined the Queensland Ambulance Service in 1959, serving in a number of Districts throughout the State and in the Central Qld. Aerial Ambulance, fully operational to Coronary Care; retired in 1993 as Assistant Commissioner, QAS., Metropolitan Region 5.
An Honorary Officer within the Education Department of the QAS.

Medal of the Order of Australia for "Service to the Community especially the Ambulance, Fire and State Emergency Services, 1992."

Granted personal Arms by the Lord Lyon King of Arms, Scotland in 1992.

Founder Member, Fellow, Past President of the Institute of Ambulance Officers (Aust.).
Fellow & Life Member of the Australian College of Ambulance Professionals.
Fellow and Life Member of Paramedics Australasia, FPA

Officer of the most Venerable Order of the Hospital of St. John of Jerusalem.

Published: 'Papers and Presentations 1975-1992' - as presented at Medical conferences and seminars on subjects of Pre-hospital Emergency Care, techniques and procedures.

Author: "Trust Me, I'm an Ambulance Officer" (1993); the writing on a brief history of the first 100 years of the Queensland Ambulance Transport Brigade to its evolution to the Queensland Ambulance Service, and the experiences of an Ambulance Officer.

Hobbies : Bonsai plants; Oil painting - landscapes.

Malcolm C. McDonald, Esq.

INDEX.

Made in the USA
Monee, IL
04 November 2026

67386694R00138